How To SWIM

AS IF YOU'RE SLEEPING

ALEX NATARE

How to Swim as if You're Sleeping by Alex Natare

The Library of Congress has cataloged this book as follows:
Natare, Alex.
How to swim as if you're sleeping/Alex Natare.

Library of Congress Control Number: 2025906112

Natare ISBN: 979-8-9927824-4-8

Author Photograph © Alex Natare

Published: Alex Natare
Bradenton, Florida 04/2025

https://www.youtube.com/@NatareSwim

Contents

Swimmer's Wish

What if you want to swim
But also want to sleep
Decided on a whim
You want the ocean's deep

But the techniques you've learned
Only how to swim fast
Once the ocean waves churned
Your session wouldn't last

If there's another way
To swim as if asleep
No matter the ocean's sway
Your strength will always keep

The water you ignore
As if you're a fish
Relaxing you might snore
A dream of swimmer's wish

What if you want to swim
But don't need to go fast
Relaxing all your limbs
It's okay to be last

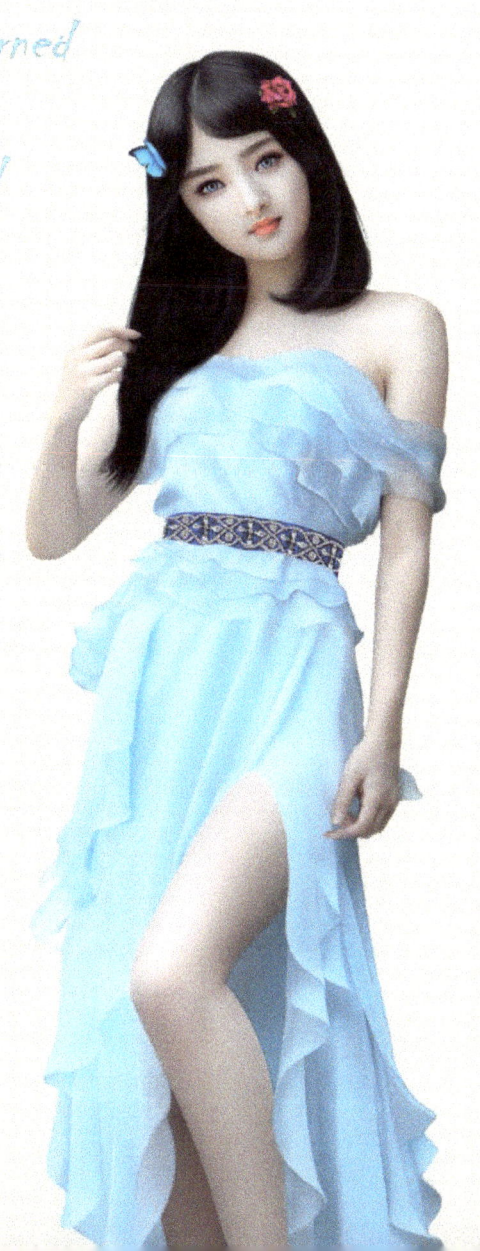

Swimming Riddle

If you want to swim like a fish,

think like a fish.

If you want to think like a fish,

think like a human.

This riddle challenges a swimmer to think like a fish and swim just as effortlessly. How can a swimmer think and swim like a fish?

How to Solve This Riddle

To solve this riddle, we must work backward from the second sentence, comparing humans to fish to understand how they think and move through the water. Since we can never truly know how a fish perceives swimming, we must rely on deductive reasoning to infer its experience. You'll find the answer near the end of this book.

Preface

While swimming in a pool, a swimming instructor took out a camera to record me. On two separate occasions, I was swimming in the ocean when someone called 911, thinking I needed to be rescued because the water conditions were too rough. I was simply swimming and didn't need to be rescued. Additionally, while swimming at the beach, I noticed beachgoers paddling out on their floaties, furtively trying to record me.

On several occasions, beachgoers approached me after seeing me swim at the beach, asking about my techniques. However, I could only give brief explanations due to time constraints. This is why I decided to write a book on how to swim. I want to provide something concrete to ensure there's no doubt that I can effectively convey my message on such an important topic.

What sets this book apart from other how-to-swim books? Typical how-to-swim books focus on swimming fast in calm bodies of water, such as pools or tranquil lakes, using precise techniques for strokes and kicks. In this context, precise techniques refer to how a swimmer executes the optimal swimming style to achieve the best possible outcome, typically for speed in a competition, without wasting any effort. This is why, in Olympic swimming competitions, all the swimmers use the same precise technique to ensure the best possible results. This book explores how to harness natural forces such as gravity and water's buoyancy through a dynamic swimming approach. Rather than emphasizing precise techniques for speed, the focus is on safety and energy conservation—essential skills for swimming in rough waters, such as ocean surf.

Think of traditional swimming techniques as a blueprint, while the techniques in this book serve as adaptable templates. To swim fast, compete, and win in the Olympics, we must follow a blueprint that focuses on optimizing technique for maximum speed. Unfortunately, not all bodies of water are as calm and controlled as a pool. Take swimming in the surf, for example. The water is constantly changing, with calm conditions often giving way to sudden, rough waves. This is why we sometimes hear stories of even great swimmers getting into trouble, carried away by rip currents at the beach.

A template swimming technique, on the other hand, can be applied in any water conditions, whether calm or rough. It would be challenging to find instructional materials that promote a 'template' approach to swimming—one that prioritizes adaptability over rigid techniques—rather than the more common 'blueprint' method focused on strict form and mechanics. Imagine wanting to learn how to swim and discovering a hidden, overgrown path that few have ventured down. Instead of concentrating on the precise details of swimming fast, we would focus more on leveraging gravity and adapting to dynamic water conditions. This path, rarely traveled, exists because very few have focused on this template technique, preferring instead to prioritize speed.

Water is not a static medium, especially in rough conditions like the surf. When the water sloshes unpredictably around us, it becomes impossible to simply optimize technique for speed. Instead, the focus should shift to stability, energy conservation, and safety.

Warnings:

While the techniques in this book can help swimmers navigate rough waters, I strongly advise against seeking such conditions out for safety reasons. Treat these techniques as a tool to use in an emergency, such as encountering a rip current. Never deliberately swim in rough waters, no matter how well-trained you are.

Introduction

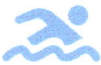

We've all heard the classic joke: 'Why did the chicken cross the road?' There are several assumptions we make about the answer. First, we assume the chicken wanted to cross the road. But what if the chicken just wanted to take a walk, and the road happened to be in the way? Second, we assume the chicken saw the road. What if the chicken was simply walking and accidentally crossed the road without noticing it? Lastly, we assume the road even existed and that a chicken crossed it. This chicken-crossing-the-road dilemma is directly related to the swimming riddle: how a swimmer should approach the water, much like how a chicken might perceive the road. This concept is the cornerstone of our how-to-swim book and will be explored later.

We'll be covering several important topics in this book. First, we'll cover mixed blessings—the challenges people face when swimming in rough water conditions, such as the surf, and how traditional swimming lessons may hinder them. Mixed Blessings also explores how our senses—such as sight, taste, hearing, and smell—can sometimes hinder our swimming abilities. Second, we'll examine breathing techniques – How to breathe properly and a method to test breathing efficiency after swimming. Third, we'll explore equilibrium – How to recuperate faster than the expenditure rate to prolong the swimming session. Fourth, we'll dive into muscle management – How to properly relax muscles while swimming to leverage gravity. Fifth, we'll cover stroking technique—how to stroke and at what angle to maximize the benefits of gravity and water's buoyancy, utilizing angular acceleration calculations. Lastly, we'll answer the swimming riddle – How to swim like a fish.

This book aims to bridge the gap between traditional swimming techniques for calm water and my approach to swimming in rougher conditions, such as the surf. Due to the recovery rate being faster than the expenditure rate while swimming and leveraging gravity—something that will be covered later—the techniques in this book can ideally be used for meditation and relaxation as if you're sleeping. Finally, we can answer why even skilled swimmers face challenges in rough water conditions, such as rip currents.

Both swimmers and non-swimmers alike will greatly benefit from this book. For non-swimmers, this book serves as an excellent starting point to learn how to swim leisurely at your own pace, in a cost-effective manner. For swimmers who have yet to tackle rough water conditions, such as those found in the surf at the beach, this book will be the key to unlocking those challenges. The way this book presents swimming techniques is unique and rarely found elsewhere. I hope readers will benefit greatly from it, just as I have enjoyed writing it.

CHAPTER 1
Challenges
of Learning
How to Swim

Knowing how to swim could save our lives one day— this is an irrefutable fact. Yet, it's baffling that 54 percent of Americans can't swim well enough to save themselves. On average, ten people drown every day[1]. If swimming is so crucial, what's preventing us from learning how to swim?

In this chapter, we'll explore the challenges people face when learning to swim. We'll ask important questions, such as 'Why do we swim?' and discuss common mistakes made in the learning process. I'll also explain how fitness relates to swimming techniques and help you assess your fitness level to ensure proper preparation. Finally, to overcome the swimming learning curve, we'll apply a divide-and-conquer approach.

Why Do We Swim?

There's no point in trying to learn how to swim if we don't understand why we want to swim in the first place. Without a clear purpose, we're likely to give up halfway through the process. In fact, most people stop swimming after grade school. Understanding why we swim is essential for not only successfully learning how to swim but also for continuing to swim into adulthood.

So, why do we want to swim? Is it to race against someone in the next lane? Is it to win a gold medal at the Olympics or swim from Cuba to Florida, or across the English Channel? Or perhaps our reason is simpler—to swim for the sake of swimming, without any ambitious goals. The material in this book focuses on swimming for relaxation and meditation by leveraging gravity, rather than for competition. If your goal is to swim competitively or across oceans, there are plenty of resources available for that. This book is about swimming to relax; therefore, it does not focus on speed, which can sometimes stress the body.

Wrong Learning Method Used

Imagine a world where there are only race cars, and no regular everyday cars. We visit dealership after dealership, and the only cars shown to us are race cars. Not knowing any better, we end up purchasing a race car for everyday driving. Since everyone else is doing the same, it seems normal and doesn't feel out of place.

Most swimmers who want to learn how to swim are not planning to race against anyone, nor are they aiming to swim in the Olympics or across the waters from Cuba to the English Channel. When we want to learn how to swim, we're often forced to follow one method, regardless of the stress it places on our bodies or the time and cost involved due to its complexity. The only approach presented is learning how to swim fast.

What if our goal is to swim for leisure— to relax and meditate, without focusing on speed? These techniques are much harder to find in the mainstream. The primary goal of this book is to help us swim in a relaxed, meditative state. Swimming fast will not be the focus of the techniques shared here. This is for those who want to swim for the sake of swimming, not for competitive aspirations.

Whether fast or slow, understanding the reason behind our desire to learn how to swim is essential. Knowing our purpose will guide us in selecting the most suitable method. Just because this book emphasizes a relaxed swimming technique doesn't mean we can't develop speed to compete. The swimming techniques discussed here can be valuable for swimmers of all skill levels and styles.

Tailor Fitness Level to Techniques

Imagine we could perform a swimming stroke and kick at the speed of light. We jump into a body of water and begin swimming. Would we swim at the speed of light or slower? Neither—we wouldn't get anywhere, because the moment we hit the water, stroking and kicking at that speed, the stress on our bodies would cause our arms and legs to shatter.

Just because someone can lift three hundred pounds at the gym doesn't mean we should attempt the same on our first time working out. If this is true for weightlifting, why shouldn't it apply to swimming as well? If we try to lift three hundred pounds at the gym on our first workout, we'll fail; then, we'll likely give up and never return. The same can be said for swimming. When someone first learns how to swim, they're often shown the same techniques that veteran swimmers use. Not only are these techniques complex, but they are also extremely difficult for beginners. Using them, beginners will become winded quickly, ruining their swimming session. This can be discouraging, and there's a high chance they will give up swimming altogether. This is where fitness level plays a crucial role in swimming techniques.

Imagine it's many years in the future, and humans have invented a knowledge transfer device that allows one person to transfer expert knowledge to another. A novice uses this device to gain the swimming knowledge of an Olympic swimmer and jumps into the pool to race against that swimmer. Despite the knowledge transfer, the Olympian would most likely still win. The reason is that the novice doesn't have the same physique or fitness level as the Olympian, who has built specific muscle strength and conditioning through years of training.

That's why it's crucial to tailor swimming techniques to each swimmer's skill level. Swimming should be enjoyable, and the last thing we want is to introduce complex maneuvers or stressful techniques. We don't want swimmers to give up, as they often do, or dread their sessions because the methods are too complicated or put too much stress on the body. After finishing this book, you should be eager to swim, rain or shine, because it will feel easy, relaxing, and fun!

Divide and Conquer

A popular saying goes, 'The whole is greater than the sum of its parts,' meaning that a system as a whole is more valuable than simply adding up each component. This is particularly true for someone learning how to swim. It can be frustrating to be expected to master all the related swimming techniques at once. To make learning how to swim easier, it's crucial to identify and analyze all the steps involved. Then, we can practice by focusing on one technique at a time, using a divide-and-conquer approach. This way, a swimmer learning to swim won't be overwhelmed by having to learn all the techniques concurrently. As the individual swimming techniques are gradually combined, the learning process will be more manageable.

What are the steps involved in swimming? First, we will outline the key swimming activities, then we'll explore them in greater detail in later sections. There are three main swimming activities: strokes, kicks, and breathing. Even with just these three, we can swim to some extent. However, other essential elements contribute to swimming such as gravity, muscle tension, and equilibrium, which may not be immediately apparent.

If we answer our phone while driving, we are no longer fully focused on the road. The same applies when learning how to swim. We are required to perform multiple activities at once—stroking a certain way, kicking with a specific technique, breathing after every third stroke, and so on. Multitasking can be difficult when you're first learning how to swim. To make it easier, try breaking down each swimming activity and focusing on them one at a time. Once you're comfortable with each activity, you can then combine them into a complete swimming session.

Mixed Blessings

Mixed blessings are when we're blessed with something positive but it hinders us in some way. There are several mixed blessings when it comes to swimming that make it difficult to swim in rough water conditions, even for experienced swimmers. Below are the water conditions posted by lifeguards at the beach. During red-flag water conditions, most swimmers will not be able to swim safely.

BEACH WARNING FLAGS

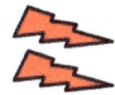

DOUBLE RED FLAGS
WATER CLOSED TO PUBLIC

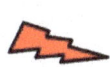

SINGLE RED FLAG
HIGH HAZARD,
HIGH SURF AND /
OR STRONG CURRENTS

MEDIUM HAZZARD
MODERATE SURF AND /
OR STRONG CURRENTS

LOW HAZARD
CALM CONDITIONS
EXERCISE CAUTIONS

FIGURE 1

There are three types of mixed blessings associated with swimming: our senses, our acquired knowledge, and our cognitive abilities. We're blessed with five well-known senses: sight, smell, taste, hearing, and touch. Additionally, we have two lesser-known senses: vestibular and proprioception. The vestibular sense is responsible for our movement and balance, providing information about the position of our head and body in space. It helps us maintain balance when sitting, standing, and walking. Proprioception, on the other hand, is the sense of body awareness. It tells us where our body parts are in relation to each other and informs us about the amount of force needed—like knowing how much pressure to apply when holding an egg without crushing it.

Contrary to popular belief, the four senses—sight, smell, taste, and hearing—hinder our swimming abilities when combined, rather than helping. We could still swim effectively if we lost any or all of these four senses. The only three senses that are truly essential for swimming are touch, vestibular, and proprioception.

When we see the water while swimming, it can trigger emotions such as fear, which increases our heart rate, consumes more oxygen, and hinders our swimming abilities. The same effect occurs if we smell, taste, or hear the water. All of these senses are heightened when we enter the water. These senses are mixed blessings because they overwhelm us— as we 'sense' too much. As a result, we become overloaded, especially as non-swimmers, when we jump into the water.

Our second mixed blessing is acquired knowledge. Many of us learned to swim through traditional lessons early in life, and the swimming techniques we've acquired are based on these lessons. This becomes a mixed blessing because we are taught to swim in a very mechanical way, with a focus on swimming fast in calm water. However, when a swimmer trained in calm water encounters rough conditions, they often try to apply the same static techniques to an ever-changing, churning body of water. This mismatch creates difficulties because the techniques we learn are not suited to the dynamic nature of rough water.

Think of it like taking a Formula 1 race car to drive on a fine-sandy beach. Not only would the driving techniques be incompatible, but we would also need a completely different car. A self-taught swimmer, on the other hand, would adapt by employing a variety of techniques suited to different water conditions. This flexibility makes a self-taught swimmer more adaptable to varying water conditions compared to someone trained with rigid swimming techniques. In this context, early swimming lessons can be a mixed blessing, as we may need to adapt traditional methods to swim effectively in rough water.

Lastly, due to our senses and some of our training, we tend to overthink while swimming. For example, when the water is rough, our senses pick up on the changes, and our thoughts process it as dangerous. Overanalyzing the situation in this way causes worry, which can overwhelm us and hinder our swimming abilities. This is one reason why a baby, just a couple of months old with lower cognitive abilities, can often learn how to swim better than an adult. Because of this, they can swim more instinctively and without the mental barriers that can hold adults back.

How to Overcome Mixed Blessings

To overcome the first mixed blessing, we need to dull the senses that aren't essential for swimming. Focus on amplifying the touch, vestibular, and proprioception senses, while tuning out the others that could overwhelm us in the water.

To overcome the second mixed blessing of prior formal swimming training, we must recognize that not all bodies of water are calm like a pool. While swimming lessons are beneficial, they may not always help when faced with rough water conditions. In these situations, the same swim-fast techniques might not be effective. We need to adjust our swimming technique based on the water environment we're in. If the water is very rough, we should avoid techniques like twisting the torso, which could lead to imbalance.

Instead, our main priorities should be conserving energy, maintaining balance, and ensuring safety.

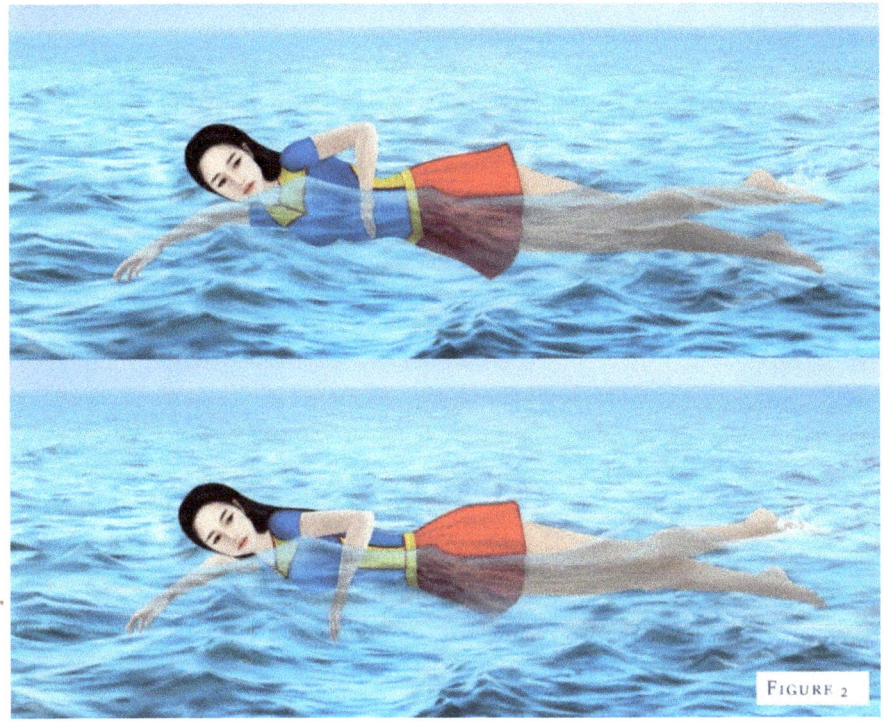

FIGURE 2

As seen with the above two swimming positions in Figure 2, the first position is tilted by 45°, and the second one is relatively flat. In rough water conditions, such as the surf, stability becomes a top priority. When we swim with a tilted body position (45° or steeper), we create a more dynamic posture that may be effective for speed and streamlined movement in calm water. However, in rough water, this position can make us more vulnerable to being tossed around by waves. The tilting of the body disrupts our balance and reduces the amount of surface area we present to the water, making it harder to maintain control.

Now, consider the second position: swimming with a relatively flat body. This position, although less dynamic, offers significantly better stability. When we keep our body closer to the surface, aligned horizontally and flat, we distribute our weight more evenly across the water. This creates a broader surface area for the water to interact with, which gives us more resistance to the waves and a higher level of balance. Think of it as trying to balance on a wide platform as opposed to a narrow one.

In rough water, this stability is crucial. The flatter swimming position allows us to better absorb the force of waves without losing control, helping to prevent us from getting off course or tiring out too quickly. Beyond balance, this position also plays a key role in energy conservation. By keeping our body flat, we use less energy trying to fight against the water's movements, allowing us to conserve stamina for longer swimming sessions. Additionally, when swimming flat, we make better use of the water's natural forces, such as buoyancy and lift, which help us stay afloat with less effort.

In essence, adopting a relatively flat position in rough water is about prioritizing control, balance, and efficiency over speed. It's a position that allows swimmers to deal with unpredictable water dynamics more safely and effectively, ensuring that energy isn't wasted and that swimmers can stay afloat for longer periods, even in challenging environments.

To overcome the third mixed blessing of our cognitive abilities, we must resist the urge to overanalyze while swimming and instead trust our instincts. While thinking critically is valuable, excessive thinking can be counterproductive. Fear, doubt, and a loss of confidence can make us inefficient swimmers, leading to unnecessary tension and wasted energy. By staying calm and managing our emotions, we can maintain a steady heart rate, which in turn allows us to swim longer and more efficiently. The key is to swim with the water, not against it—working in harmony with its natural flow rather than resisting it.

For those who fear swimming or water in general, logic and reason can help overcome these insecurities. For example, if you're 6 feet tall and the water is only 4 feet deep, simply standing up will allow you to breathe naturally. Additionally, if you jump into the water and struggle against it instead of working with it, you'll use up oxygen much faster. By applying logical reasoning, we can build confidence, reduce heart rate, and conserve air—leading to a more controlled and enjoyable swimming experience.

CHAPTER II

Swimming Foundations

Swimming foundations consist of three main elements: strokes, kicks, and breathing. In this chapter, we'll first compare swimming to everyday activities like walking, providing a familiar point of reference for swimmers. Then, we'll explore stroke techniques, focusing on the optimal elbow and arm angles. Next, we'll examine the role of kicking in maintaining balance and positioning. Finally, we'll discuss breathing techniques and the crucial role of air in swimming.

Swimming Assessment

Before diving into the details of swimming, it's important to conduct a preliminary assessment to understand why certain techniques maximize relaxation and minimize stress. The best way to do this is by examining familiar activities—like walking—to use as a basis for comparison. What similarities exist between walking and swimming when it comes to relaxation?

One of the most natural activities we do is walking. When we walk in a relaxed state, we don't consciously think about our strides or arm swings—they happen automatically. However, the moment we start focusing on them, we disrupt the natural rhythm. This concept is similar to physics, where observing a subject can alter its behavior. Likewise, when we overanalyze our strides or arm movements, our walking becomes less fluid and more forced, making it feel unnatural and less relaxed.

The walking exercise we just did mirrors the principles of swimming. The most natural and relaxed way to swim is by letting go of the conscious effort—essentially, by not overthinking the fact that we're swimming. The moment we start focusing too much on our strokes and kicks, we disrupt our natural rhythm. For instance, we may instinctively start kicking faster, extending our arms unnaturally, or altering our body position in ways that create unnecessary strain. Since these adjustments are not natural, they can lead to discomfort or even stress. In the following sections, we'll explore how to find the most comfortable swimming position. Because comfort levels vary from person to person, we'll conduct tests to help each individual determine their optimal swimming technique.

Straight or Bent Arm?

Should we swim with our arms straight or slightly bent? To answer this, we first need to ask ourselves: Are we aiming for speed, or do we want to swim in a relaxed, natural state? Extending the arm straight while swimming is common, particularly among experienced swimmers who have the upper body strength to maintain this technique. However, for beginners learning to swim for the first time, a straight arm can be challenging and even discouraging, as it requires significant upper body strength. While a veteran swimmer may find it effortless, a beginner might struggle and risk giving up altogether. In this section, we'll explore whether swimming with a straight arm or a slight bend is more conducive to a relaxed and comfortable swimming experience.

Before we begin, let's consider a hypothetical scenario to illustrate whether a straight or bent arm is better for relaxed swimming. Imagine two rods—one straight and one slightly curved. Using common sense, we know that a curved rod can withstand stress more effectively than a straight one due to its structural integrity. The same principle applies to swimming. Extending our arms straight during a stroke places more strain on the muscles while bending them slightly helps maintain a more natural and supportive structure, reducing stress and promoting relaxation.

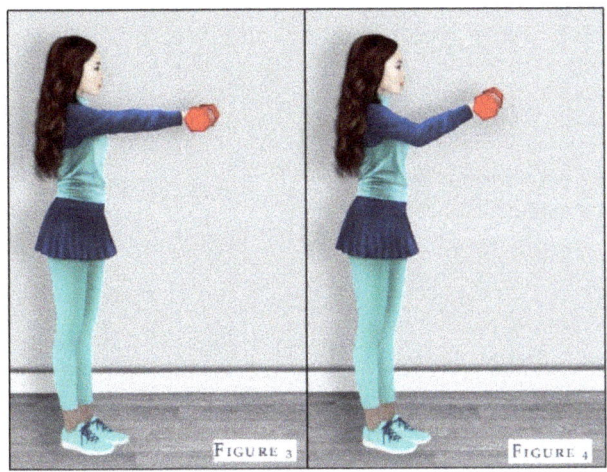

FIGURE 3 FIGURE 4

To illustrate this concept, let's start by standing up straight and facing forward, as shown in Figure 3. Extend one arm straight out parallel to the ground with the palm facing upward. To speed up the exercise, imagine holding about five pounds of weight in your hand. How long could you maintain this position?

For step two, repeat the same motion, but bend your elbow and bring your arm closer to your body, as shown in Figure 4. How long could you hold position one versus position two? Even without physically performing the exercise, we can intuitively tell that bending the arm feels more comfortable, and it can be maintained for a longer time.

From this, we can conclude that swimming with bent arms is more relaxing and less stressful than swimming with straight arms extended. Bending the arms allows us to swim longer with less strain, ultimately helping us conserve energy.

Some may argue that swimming with straight arms allows you to gather more water, which can help you swim faster. However, since the goal here is to relax and swim with minimal stress, a bent arm is a more effective option. A bent arm not only reduces strain but also promotes a more comfortable and sustainable swimming experience. Additionally, when swimming in rough conditions, such as at the beach among the surf, having bent arms adds stability and provides a safer alternative, as it helps maintain better control in the water.

Arm/Elbow Angle

Based on the previous exercise, swimming with bent arms is optimal for relaxation and stress reduction. However, the degree of arm bend is also crucial. If we bend our arms too little, our stroke can still cause strain. On the other hand, bending them too much will reduce the effectiveness of our stroke. The key is finding a middle ground—a moderate bend—that offers the best balance between reducing stress, maintaining stability, and ensuring that our stroke remains effective in propelling us forward.

We can perform several exercises to find the optimal arm/ elbow angle while swimming. A simple test is to swim and gradually adjust the arm/elbow angle throughout the swim. Start with a comfortable angle, then slowly increase or decrease it as you go. When the angle becomes too small and uncomfortable, adjust it again until your arms are straightened. By repeating this process, you can determine the most comfortable and effective arm/elbow angle for your swim.

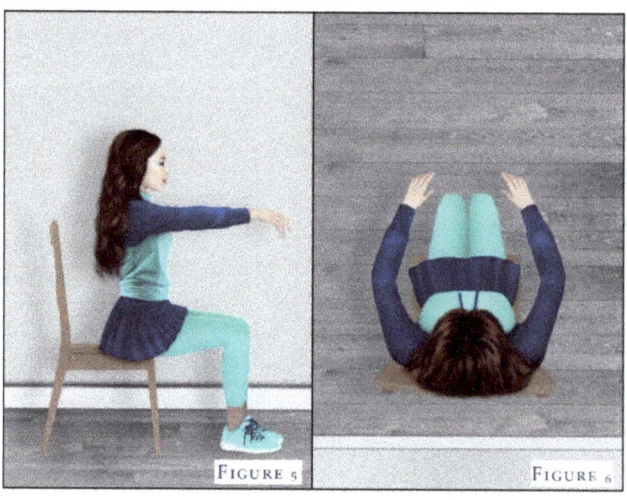

FIGURE 5   FIGURE 6

Another simple test is to find a chair and sit comfortably. Then, raise both arms in front of you, with your palms drooping down, about shoulder height parallel to the ground as shown in Figures 5 and 6. This mirrors the starting position before executing a swim stroke. There are no strict rules for how straight or bent the arm should be during the stroke. Depending on your comfort level and fitness, you can choose to extend the arm straight or bend it slightly. If speed is the goal, extend the arm fully during the stroke, but if comfort and relaxation are your priority, bend the arm slightly.

Imagine swimming like the pedaling motion involved in riding a bike, but instead of spinning the arms in a circle, you draw an elliptical shape with your hands and forearms. The key is not to use the palm to gather water but to initiate the stroke starting from the wrist upward toward the shoulder. Using the palm to gather water, especially during prolonged and repeated strokes, places unnecessary stress on the wrist.

Kicking Techniques

Kicking provides stability, body positioning, and propulsion while swimming. While it might seem like a simple concept, if kicking were truly that straightforward, everyone would be a proficient swimmer. There's much more to a swim kick than meets the eye. If we remove speed from the equation, we can evaluate the importance of kicking in relation to the three major swimming activities: stroke, breathing, and kicking.

When it comes to swimming, having good breathing technique is the most essential element. No matter how skilled a swimmer may be, once they run out of air, their swim session is over. This leaves kicking and stroking to be ranked in terms of importance. While the swim kick is crucial for propulsion, it's inefficient if you want to conserve energy. Swimming freestyle while kicking can consume up to 75% more oxygen than swimming with just the arms[2]. The arm swim stroke contributes approximately 90% to the swimming velocity among elite swimmers[5]. Given these statistics, the swim stroke ranks second in importance, while the swim kick ranks last when it comes to conserving energy for efficient swimming.

If the swim kick ranks last among the three main foundations of swimming and consumes up to 75% more oxygen than the arm stroke alone, should we still use it while swimming? For competitive swimmers, the answer is yes — they should continue practicing and using kicking techniques to propel themselves forward. However, if the goal is to relax and meditate while swimming, kicking should primarily focus on providing stability and proper body positioning. There's no need to worry about intricate kicking techniques in this case.

How should we approach kicking for stability and body positioning? The best approach is for each swimmer to sense it by feel. Once the swimmer has found their rhythm, they can kick whenever they feel the need or to maintain balance. Although there's no strict requirement for a specific kicking rhythm, it might be helpful to suggest a simple kicking pattern until the swimmer becomes comfortable and can adjust it to their preferences later on.

To establish a rhythm, try kicking in sync with your strokes. When the right arm performs the stroke, kick with the right foot, and do the same with the left arm and foot. Alternate like this, and your kick will fall into place. Logically, bending your knees too much can create drag. Drag is the friction caused by water interacting with your body, slowing you down while swimming. With this in mind, I recommend you kick, but avoid bending your knees excessively. This approach is straightforward, which is exactly what we're aiming for. After all, the goal is to relax and meditate while swimming, not to be bogged down by complex techniques.

Since kicking consumes up to 75% more oxygen than a stroke, we can try to reduce kicking in general. Instead of kicking with every arm stroke, we can reduce the kick rate to once every two arm strokes or only kick when balancing or positioning is required. If kicking isn't necessary for stability, we can reduce it even further, depending on how well we can maintain balance. Keep in mind that if we stop kicking altogether, our legs will sink, and we'll begin swimming almost vertically, which resembles treading water. Ultimately, we'll kick primarily to maintain balance, or if we have plenty of oxygen reserves, we can kick whenever we feel like it.

Breathing Technique – Overview

Breathing technique is more important than kicking or stroking because, without proper air management, a swimmer will quickly become exhausted and unable to continue. Since proper breathing is the foundation of swimming, mastering this technique should be the top priority. Once the breathing technique is proficient, the swimmer can then focus on integrating strokes and kicks into their swim routine. Swimmers should aim to breathe in the same natural way as they do while walking on land. This doesn't mean breathing slowly like on land, but the process of acquiring and processing air should feel similar. There should never be a shortness of breath—swimming should feel as relaxed as a leisurely walk. If a swimmer feels winded or is struggling to catch their breath, it's a sign they're exerting too much effort or improperly managing air. In that case, they should slow down and return to a relaxed, steady breathing pattern, similar to how they would breathe while walking.

There are many misconceptions about the level of fitness required to be able to swim. Imagine walking leisurely on land—do you need to be fit to walk slowly and comfortably? Swimming can feel even more relaxed than walking, as your body weight is supported by the water. People often experience shortness of breath because their technique and effort level don't align with their fitness level while swimming. With proper technique and the right effort, a swimmer can breathe just as easily in the water as they would while walking on land even with differing fitness levels.

Only exhale slowly when your nose and mouth are underwater. When your head is turned to the side and your nose and mouth are above the water, take a quick breath in. Exhaling while your nose and mouth are above the water wastes valuable seconds that could be better spent inhaling.

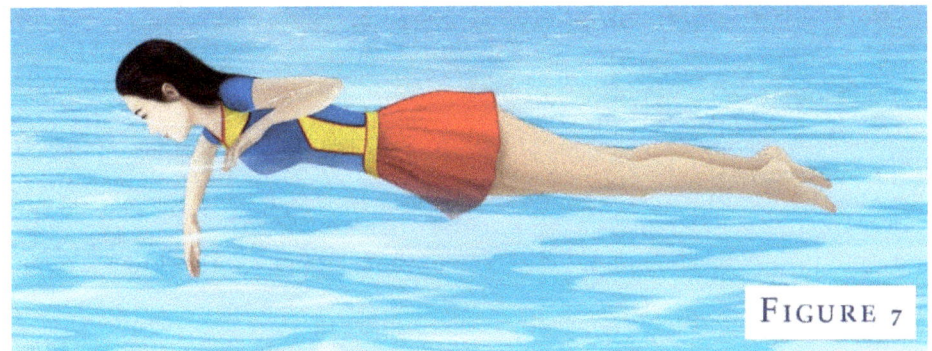

When nose and mouth are underwater, continuously exhale slowly.

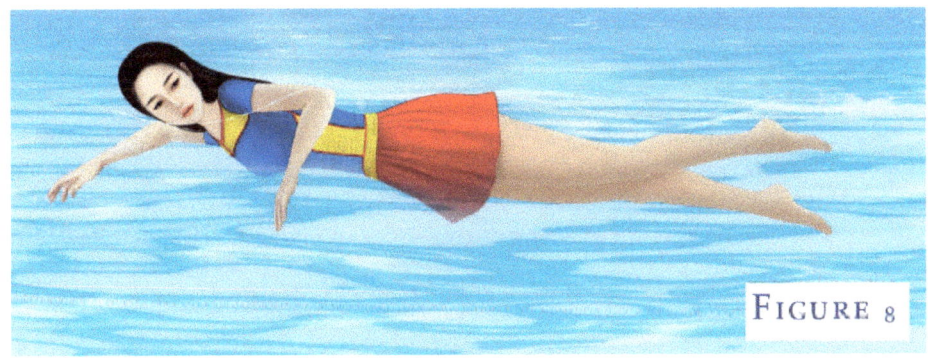

Turn the head sideways and inhale fast.

Exhaling properly is more important than inhaling while swimming. Our body converts oxygen into carbon dioxide, which is then released into our lungs. Even if we try to inhale more air, if our lungs are already filled with carbon dioxide, the amount of oxygen we take in will be minimal. This leads to oxygen deprivation, making swimming difficult or impossible. Since we quickly inhale when our nose and mouth are above water, we invariably spend more time exhaling than inhaling.

It's also important to clear our lungs of carbon dioxide periodically, even when using the proper breathing technique. When we quickly inhale air while swimming, the oxygen-to-carbon dioxide ratio in our lungs can become unbalanced. At this point, a swimmer should slow down and consciously force out the air, perhaps by coughing, to reset the lungs at intervals. Once this is done, the swimmer can resume swimming until the next necessary carbon dioxide air reset.

Breathing Technique – Detailed Explanations

When transitioning from land to water, the air in your lungs is in a normal mix. As you begin swimming and performing strokes, your body starts to consume oxygen. Once your head is submerged, begin exhaling slowly at a moderate pace while simultaneously turning your head to prepare for inhaling. Avoid forcefully expelling the air; aim for a steady, controlled exhale. As you approach the end of your exhale, your nose and mouth should be just about to clear the water's surface. Once your nose and mouth are above the water, quickly inhale air, then turn your head back into the water to continue the breathing cycle.

Sometimes, simply turning the head sideways may not be enough to lift the nose and mouth above the water for breathing. When swimming fast, the head moves through the water and displaces it, creating a pocket of air behind the head for breathing. However, when a swimmer is still learning and swimming at a slower pace, this water displacement may not occur. To compensate for this, use the leverage of the arm pushing down at that moment when stroking to help keep the nose and mouth above the water, facilitating better inhalation.

A common issue for swimmers when attempting to inhale is accidentally breathing in water. If done correctly, no water should be inhaled, as water is denser than air. Swimmers should aim to strike a balance between inhaling quickly and avoiding pulling in water. With practice, this can be mastered. However, it's important to acknowledge that, especially in rough or unpredictable conditions, water can occasionally enter the mouth. When this happens, it typically stays at the front of the mouth, so be prepared to expel it promptly.

Avoid overcompensating when breathing while swimming. Only turn your head sideways to inhale, keeping the upper body steady. Inhale quickly, then turn your head back down to exhale and continue swimming.

Breathing while swimming is a bit different from breathing on land. Since only a brief moment is available to inhale, it's natural to breathe in quickly rather than slowly. This is just the starting point, but over time, a rhythm or cycle can form, such as breathing in after every third stroke. Each time the arm stroke goes down, the leverage from the arm can help raise the head to breathe.

Breathe in similar to the bottom image of Figure 2 (below).

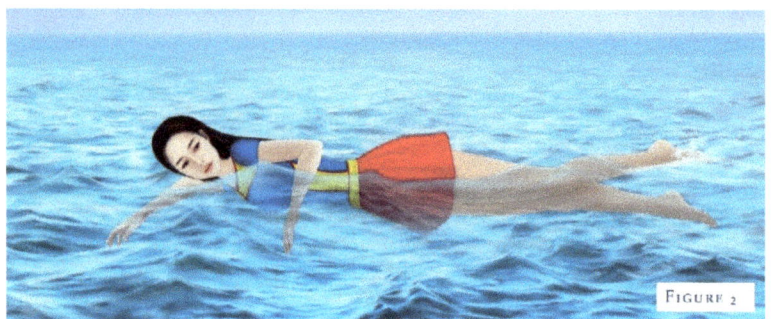

The goal of breathing while swimming is to make it as natural as possible, similar to breathing on land. When combined with the equilibrium concept discussed in a later chapter, this breathing technique will feel as effortless as walking, allowing swimmers to cover long distances without running out of breath. Once fully mastered, this technique will be particularly useful when navigating more challenging water conditions, such as swimming in the surf.

One breathing technique involves holding the breath while swimming, but this is not recommended. As mentioned earlier, the body converts oxygen into carbon dioxide, and if a swimmer holds their breath for too long, they will quickly run out of oxygen and be unable to continue swimming. While this technique may work for experienced swimmers, it is not recommended for beginners.

Constantly breathing in and out ensures that the air in the lungs stays fresh, similar to breathing and relaxing on land. Not everyone has the same fitness level, so holding their breath while swimming might not be feasible for everyone. For example, just because an expert free diver like Herbert Nitsch can dive to 253 meters doesn't mean the average person can. Similarly, just because an expert swimmer can hold their breath while swimming doesn't mean that an average swimmer can do the same.

CHAPTER III
Swimming Concepts

The previous chapter covered the three main foundations of swimming, along with their rankings and importance. In this chapter, we will delve into the concepts that tie these foundations together and explore how they relate to one another as a whole. We'll examine muscle management during strokes and kicks and how they engage the muscles of the entire body. Additionally, we'll discuss how rhythm management can improve swimming efficiency for relaxation, and how the concept of equilibrium can enhance endurance during longer swimming sessions.

Muscle Management

If we closely observe someone swimming and try to duplicate their motions, will we be able to swim like them? While swimming motions are an important part of the equation, they are only one piece of the larger swimming puzzle. Beneath those motions lies the way we manage and engage our muscles while swimming. Simply copying someone's swim motions without understanding how to properly manage and utilize the muscles can result in an ineffective swim and potentially lead to injury.

We've established that swimming with bent arms is optimal for relaxation and stress reduction, but what about muscle management? How should we engage our muscles while performing strokes or kicks? To determine the best way to manage muscle use, we can revisit the same exercise we used to compare bent and straight arms. This will help us find the most efficient way to use our muscles while swimming.

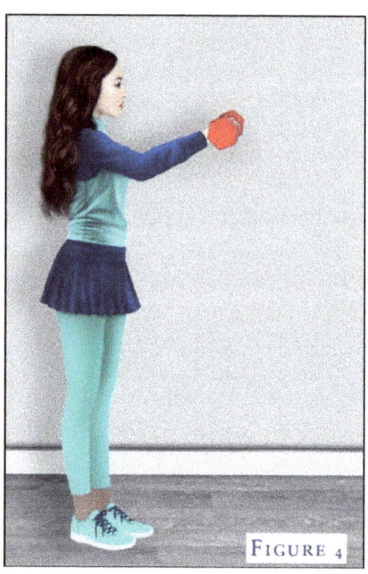

FIGURE 4

Extend the arm out, as shown in Figure 4, with a slight bend while holding a 5 lb. weight. In the first part, focus primarily on using the muscles of the arm. Then, try again, but this time engage the arm muscles along with the upper body muscles, working as a continuous unit. Next, incorporate the core muscles into the movement. Finally, bring all of the body's muscles together, using them as a single, unified unit.

We should begin to notice the pattern here. Although we're swimming with our arms to perform a stroke, it's essential to engage the entire body's muscles to work in harmony with the arms, creating one continuous, functioning unit. Relying solely on the arm muscles can lead to unnecessary stress and is not ideal for prolonged swimming sessions.

The same principle applies to our kicks. If we kick using only the leg muscles, the outcome will be similar to stroking with just the arm muscles—ineffective and stressful. Instead, we should combine the leg muscles with the core muscles while kicking. Even better, our entire body's muscles should work together in an interconnected way during the kick. While this requires some effort, it's crucial to stay relaxed, even while using the whole body's muscles as a unified unit during swimming.

The key takeaway from this section is that although a stroke or kick may seem to primarily involve the arm or leg muscles, it's essential to engage the entire body's muscles instead. All the muscles should work together, interconnected, never isolated. If we disconnect the arm and shoulder muscles from the rest of the body's muscles while swimming, we'll lose a significant amount of strength. Always aim to connect and use your body's muscles as one cohesive unit. It's like pedaling a bike: the front wheel is connected to the back, both connected by a chain, which in turn connects to our feet as we pedal. The moment we disconnect any part of that system, it all falls apart. While using your muscles as a unified force in swimming, it's equally important to stay relaxed. Tension during swimming doesn't help—it only disrupts performance and creates unnecessary strain.

Rhythm Management

Maintaining a consistent rhythm is essential for any swimming technique. To truly enjoy a swim session, we should stop focusing on our strokes, kicks, breathing, or all the complex motions involved. Once we establish a natural rhythm, swimming becomes as effortless and relaxing as walking on land. Over time, swimming will no longer feel like a chore, but rather a pleasant activity that we look forward to with each opportunity.

There are two types of rhythm that swimmers can establish. One is a basic rhythm that can be used by everyone, while the other is tailored to the individual swimmer's preferences. For example, if someone is left-handed, they shouldn't be expected to perform tasks suited for right-handed individuals. We'll first explore the basic rhythm, then delve into how swimmers can adjust their rhythm to fit their personal preferences.

Let's start with the basic rhythm for our strokes. Imagine our swimming stroke for the left and right arms as two people sitting on opposite ends of a see-saw. When the right arm pushes down on the water, the left arm rises, and when the left arm pushes down, the right arm rises. Our shoulders act like the ends of the see-saw—when one shoulder tilts slightly down, the other tilts slightly up. This motion helps leverage the body for breathing. While this body tilt is a natural movement, a swimmer may choose to adjust it based on personal preferences.

Let's explore breathing rhythm where swimmers can apply their preferences. Some swimmers may choose to breathe on just one side (single side), while others may alternate and breathe on both sides (bilateral). If a swimmer feels comfortable breathing only on the left or right side, that's perfectly fine. There are pros and cons to each approach. Breathing on one side is generally easier to learn and can be favored depending on whether the swimmer is left- or right-handed. This method works well for those who swim for one to two hours a day. However, for swimmers who train for longer distances, like four or more hours per day, learning bilateral breathing may be more beneficial. It helps balance the body's rotation and prevents excessive soreness on one side.

The rhythm for the kick is quite simple. As mentioned earlier, you can kick and stroke on the same side simultaneously. If the left arm is stroking, then kick with the left foot, and do the same for the right arm and foot. However, if this feels uncomfortable, try alternating and performing a left-arm-right foot combo, where you stroke with the left arm and kick with the right foot at the same time. Then, alternate by stroking with the right arm and kicking with the left foot. Additionally, since kicking consumes up to 75% more oxygen than stroking, it's best to use kicking primarily for balance and positioning, rather than propulsion. Our goal is to swim comfortably and adjust to the water conditions. For example, if swimming in the ocean surf where waves are crashing to one side, it might be a good idea to breathe only on the opposite side to avoid water rushing into the mouth.

This concludes rhythm management, which is quite simple to learn. Our ultimate goal is not to get bogged down with techniques but to learn them and then forget about them. We should strive to perform swimming motions effortlessly, allowing ourselves to stay as relaxed as possible—almost as though we were sleeping. Just like a fish swimming in the water doesn't consciously think about breathing or flapping its fins every few seconds, we should strive to swim naturally, without rigid patterns. That's the ideal we should work towards.

Equilibrium

How to Swim Indefinitely

While this chapter discusses the concept of swimming indefinitely, we must acknowledge that nothing truly lasts forever. Therefore, the equilibrium swimming technique covered here is purely theoretical and should not be taken literally. We can't completely control fatigue or soreness, as we will inevitably need rest or sleep. However, if a swimmer's recovery rate exceeds or matches their expenditure rate, they could, in theory, swim indefinitely. In this context, recovery rate refers to cumulative recovery, which includes factors such as fatigue, oxygen or air consumption, soreness, and energy conservation.

If we were to clone a person for a marathon race and have one jog slowly while the other sprints, we would logically expect the one who jogs to finish the race, while the sprinter would likely be unable to sustain their pace. The jogger can finish the marathon because their recovery rate matches or exceeds their energy expenditure rate. While the sprinter's body also recovers, their energy expenditure rate exceeds their recovery rate, preventing them from completing the marathon.

Just like jogging a marathon, we also recover while swimming. The most important aspect of recovery is to manage air consumption. The moment we fall behind on air recovery, we stop swimming. In addition to air consumption and recovery, swimmers also need to recover energy by replenishing the body's fuel stores. If the body runs out of fuel or if fuel consumption exceeds the rate of recovery, coupled with insufficient sleep or rest, fatigue will set in.

As the saying goes, "An ounce of prevention is worth a pound of cure." In this case, the best way to recover energy is to avoid expending it unnecessarily. A key part of energy conservation is not using 100 percent effort when applying downward force during a stroke, but rather leveraging gravity. By relaxing and allowing the arm to fall with the downward applied force, a swimmer can save energy with every stroke. We'll explore the concept of gravity in swimming further in the next section.

Another aspect of the equilibrium concept is avoiding maximum effort while swimming. This is similar to the difference between jogging and sprinting—sprinting requires maximum effort, while jogging allows for more endurance. It's important to leave some wiggle room during a swim, especially in case of rough water conditions or muscle cramps. By maintaining a sustainable effort, we ensure we can recover safely and continue swimming without overexertion.

Gravity-Assisted Swimming

The consensus in the swimming world is to disregard gravity, as buoyancy in water counteracts its effects. However, we can unconventionally harness gravity to enhance our swim stroke. Aside from breathing, the swim stroke itself is the most crucial element of swimming technique. Since the way we use our arms while swimming is pivotal, we'll focus on optimizing arm movement to improve overall swimming efficiency. For a more in-depth understanding and calculations of gravity-assisted swimming, please refer to Appendix A (Effect of Gravity While Swimming).

What forces act on a swimmer's arm while swimming? First, gravity comes into play. When we lift our arm, gravity pulls it back down. Second, air pressure affects the arm as well. While gravity pulls the arm downward, air pressure pushes against it from all directions. Although air pressure decreases with elevation, for swimming, we can ignore it because the distance our arm travels is minimal. Third, buoyancy is a factor. As our arm moves through the water, it works against the buoyant force of the water, leading to energy expenditure. For this discussion, we will set aside considerations of air pressure and drag (resistance encountered as the swimmer moves through the water).

Once our arm is underwater and we attempt to lift it out, buoyancy comes into play, trying to push the arm upward. The water's resistance fights the motion, making it harder to lift the arm without using significant energy. However, the most important force we can control is the muscle tension in our arms. By properly managing this muscle tension, along with leveraging gravity and buoyancy, we can conserve energy and swim much more efficiently with less effort. The following sections will explain how gravity can be harnessed to assist us while swimming.

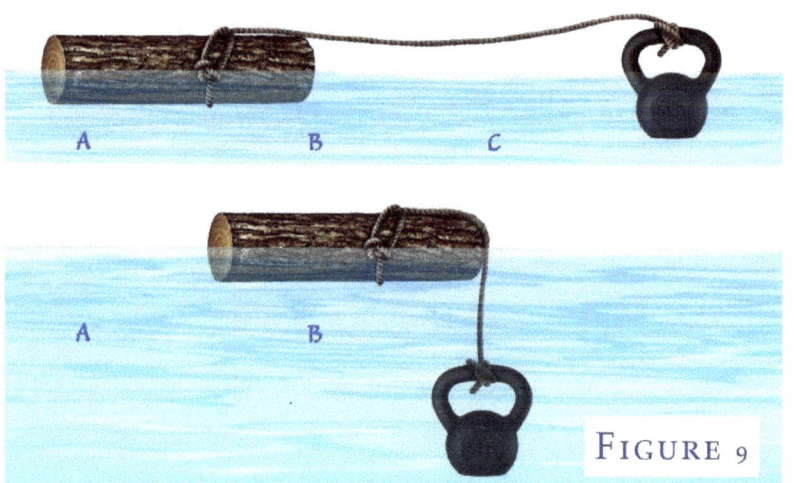

FIGURE 9

Imagine tying a rope to a log at one end and attaching a weighted object to the other end, holding the weighted object parallel to the surface of the water, as shown in Figure 9. When the weighted object is released into the water, the log should theoretically move past position B, depending on the mass of both the log and the weighted object. The combination of gravity and buoyancy would work together to move the log forward, with no energy expenditure required from an external source.

We've discussed how gravity and buoyancy can propel an object forward without expending energy, but how does this apply to swimming? Out of the three forces acting on our arms—gravity, buoyancy, and muscle tension—muscle tension plays a crucial role when we consider both gravity and buoyancy. By managing the tension in our muscles, we can leverage the effects of gravity and buoyancy to move more efficiently through the water. Instead of working against these forces, we can use them to our advantage, minimizing unnecessary energy expenditure and enhancing our ability to swim longer distances with less effort.

In the example above with the log, rope, and weighted object in the pool, each time the weighted object is released, it moves the log forward by a small amount. By continuously repeating this process, the log will gradually move across the pool without any effort or energy exerted by us to push it downward into the water. This illustrates how gravity and buoyancy, when utilized correctly, can propel an object forward without the need for physical force, allowing us to conserve energy while swimming. By applying this same concept to swimming, we can move through the water more efficiently with less effort.

To take full advantage of gravity as a free source of downward force, we should keep our arms as relaxed as possible while swimming. By reducing the muscle tension in our arms to a necessary minimum, we can maximize the use of the downward force of gravity. In this relaxed state, the only forces that should be acting on our arms during the swimming motion are gravity, buoyancy, and the force of our arm pushing down in the water.

During swimming, there are two scenarios concerning our arms:

1. Your arm pushing downward

Swimmer's arm downward force

+ Gravity

- Buoyancy

- Muscle tension

= Actual swimmer's arm downward force

FIGURE 10

2. Your arm lifting up for next stroke

Swimmer's arm uplift force

- Gravity

+ Buoyancy

- Muscle tension

= Actual swimmer's arm uplift force

FIGURE 11

A crucial factor to consider when lifting the arms for the next stroke is buoyancy. If we lift our arms above the water, buoyancy becomes zero, meaning no upward force is helping us. To take full advantage of buoyancy, we should lift the arms just enough to be above the water's surface. This minimizes drag while allowing us to benefit from the buoyant force that helps keep the arm elevated.

As shown in the equations, the forces we can directly control with our arms are our upward and downward force and muscle tension. The most efficient way to swim with our arms is to reduce muscle tension to a minimum, enabling gravity and buoyancy to do much of the work. Let's perform more calculations to understand how significant this benefit can be when swimming.

Research has shown that the weight of one arm is approximately 5 percent of a person's total body weight[3]. For example, if a person weighs 200 pounds, their arm would weigh around 10 pounds.

The key point here is that gravity can provide an assist in the downward motion of the arm during swimming. Since muscle tension and the natural resistance of connective tissues and bones will inevitably require some force to move the arm, a perfectly relaxed arm won't be able to utilize the full 10-pound weight of the arm due to the necessary muscle activation to maintain control and movement.

However, even a little increase—let's say, just 1 pound of effective downward force aided by gravity—can make a noticeable difference in energy conservation. Over time, this small energy saving can compound significantly, particularly over long swimming sessions. By reducing muscle tension to a minimum and relying on gravity, swimmers can improve efficiency, reduce fatigue, and extend their endurance. This highlights the importance of managing muscle tension and leveraging gravity, even if only partially, for optimal swimming technique.

Gaining just 1 pound of weight per stroke can make a significant difference during a long swimming session. Let's assume an average swimmer completes 60 strokes per minute. This results in an additional 60 pounds of weight pushed downward each minute or 3,600 pounds (1.8 tons) per hour. Over a two-hour session, this amounts to an extra 7,200 pounds (3.6 tons) of downward force, helping to propel the swimmer with minimal effort.

One pound is just a conservative estimate. If done correctly, this could add at least two extra pounds of weight per stroke or 120 pounds per minute. Over two hours, if we add two pounds of weight per stroke, the total extra weight amounts to 14,400 pounds or 7.2 tons. This is an astonishing amount of additional weight saved through the downstroke during a swimming session. This explains why some swimmers can swim continuously for hours. They don't feel exhausted because the energy they regain with the help of gravity exceeds the energy they expend while swimming.

To apply this method effectively, we need to understand a bit about math, geometry, gravity, and physics. Based on the angular acceleration calculations in Appendix A, the maximum force is achieved when the arm stroke begins at a position parallel to the water in front of the swimmer. This aligns with common sense as well. From that point, the swimmer should apply the swimming stroke force following the diminishing return slope outlined in Appendix A. The greatest force should be applied at a 0° angle, gradually decreasing as the stroke progresses downward into the water.

To determine the ideal angle at which to end the stroke, we need to consider how gravity influences our arm position. Without any calculations, we can observe that when the arm is pointing straight down (at a 90° angle from the body toward below), gravity is no longer assisting. Continuing the stroke beyond this point means we're working against gravity. At around 45°, the swimmer should begin to wrap up the stroke. Any further effort past this point becomes inefficient, as shown in the angular acceleration graph in Appendix A. This is the recovery phase, where the swimmer prepares for the next stroke.

The faster we swim, the more muscle tension is required to keep the arm up during each stroke. As a result, the benefits of gravity are reduced at higher speeds. With practice, we'll find the optimal swimming speed that allows us to go fast while still taking advantage of gravity, helping us conserve energy and avoid fatigue.

The gravity-assisted swimming technique is especially valuable in rough waters. A 'one-size-fits-all' technique that works in a pool won't be effective in the ocean, where waves constantly shift and crash. Mastering gravity-assisted swimming is crucial for lasting in these challenging conditions. We'll delve into this further when we explore ocean swimming.

CHAPTER IV
Time for a Swim

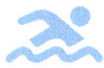

In this chapter, we will cover detailed swimming techniques, how to swim efficiently in the pool, the fitness required for swimming in the surf, and how to navigate the challenges of ocean swimming. To fully benefit from this chapter, it's essential that you first thoroughly read and understand the previous topics. We'll be using terms like *gravity-assisted swimming*, which we introduced earlier.

The pool is the ideal starting point for learning to swim because it offers a safe environment, often with a lifeguard present. The water is generally calm, and the pool's markings provide helpful guidance for swimmers. In contrast, swimming in the ocean presents more serious challenges. That's why we have a separate section dedicated to preparing swimmers and assessing their fitness before they venture into ocean swimming.

Detailed Swimming Movements

In the previous sections, including the appendices, we've covered the essential details of swimming. In this section, we'll focus on general swimming techniques. We use the term "general" to avoid getting stuck in a rigid swimming pattern, particularly given the dynamic challenges posed by rough water conditions.

Specific swimming techniques are ideal for calm waters, speed, and competition, where maximizing and minimizing efficiency is key. However, when facing dynamic, rough water, a more flexible and general approach is necessary. How should a swimmer position their arms, regulate their breathing, and adjust their kick in such conditions? While all three techniques are important, we'll primarily focus on the swimmer's strokes and breathing, as kicking is mostly used for balance in these situations.

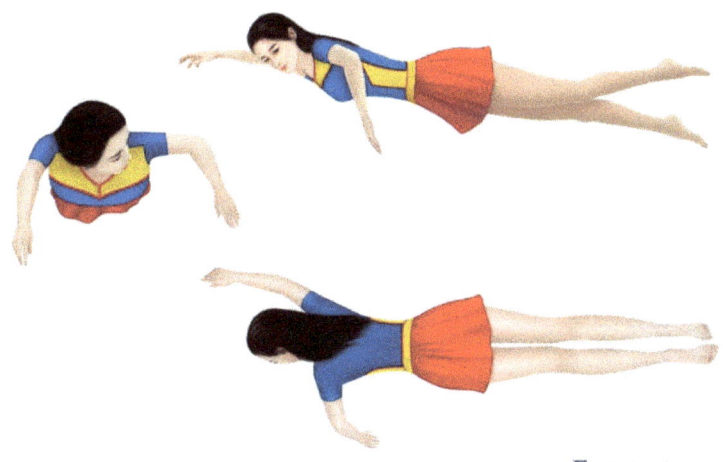

FIGURE 12

Start by taking a deep breath before swimming. Extend the right arm out parallel to the water, resting on top. Make a slight hop to bring the legs up so the body is now parallel to the water's surface. Ensure the arm is bent, as described in previous sections. The left arm can hang loose behind the shoulder. At this point, the head begins to turn left to begin breathing in, but you are still exhaling. According to the angular acceleration calculations, this is the optimal position to generate the most stroke force with the assistance of gravity.

As the arm progresses down, the angular acceleration will diminish, reaching zero at 90°. To maximize the efficiency of our swimming stroke, we should align our stroke with the diminishing return of angular acceleration. This means that when the arm is parallel to the water, we apply the most downward force.

As the stroke progresses and the angle approaches 90°, we gradually reduce the downward force, eventually ceasing the stroking force altogether.

Remember, our goal is not speed but comfort and leisure. Swimming with the palm may be effective for speed, but it can place excessive strain on the wrist over time. To avoid this, focus on initiating the stroke from the wrist upward, rather than pushing with the palm. Keep the palm relaxed and slightly drooping while performing the stroke to reduce pressure on the wrist.

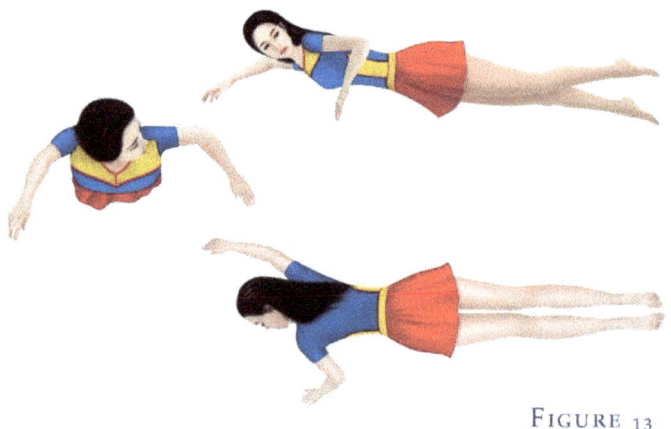

FIGURE 13

Continue the right arm stroke downward, with a slight outward motion. This subtle outward movement creates a more natural stroke compared to a straight-down motion, which feels less fluid. Keep the arm relaxed, allowing all muscles to work in harmony as a continuous unit. Maximize stroke strength in alignment with the angular acceleration curve, and complete the stroke just beyond 45°. By this point, the head should have fully rotated to the left, with the nose and mouth above the water. This is the moment to take a quick, deep breath, inhaling swiftly.

Depending on your swimming proficiency and comfort level, as well as the water conditions (calm or choppy), you may need to slightly tilt your body toward the side you're breathing on. To gain leverage for this tilt, use the arm that's currently stroking to consciously push down on the water. This will provide the necessary support to tilt your body or even raise your head above the water to check your surroundings, such as buoy markers or landmarks when swimming in the ocean.

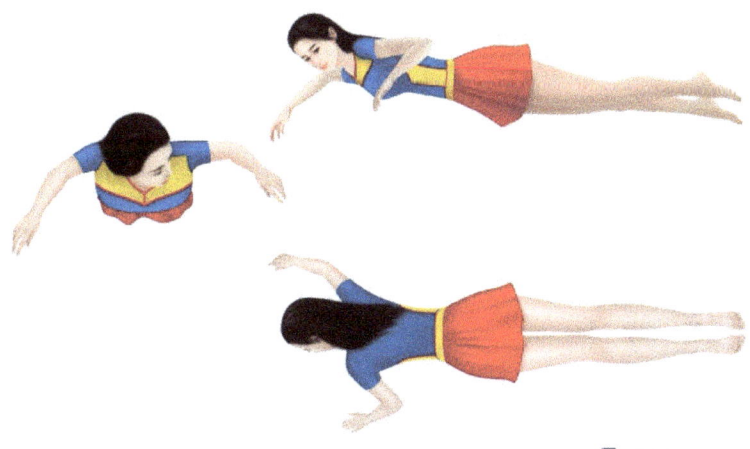

FIGURE 14

Continue to stroke downward with the right arm, angling it slightly outward. Meanwhile, the left arm is preparing for the next stroke. Once you've finished taking a quick breath, your head should begin turning back down into the water. At this point, start exhaling slowly. As emphasized in the previous section on breathing, a swimmer should never hold their breath. You should either inhale quickly when your nose and mouth are above the water or exhale slowly and continuously when your face is back in the water.

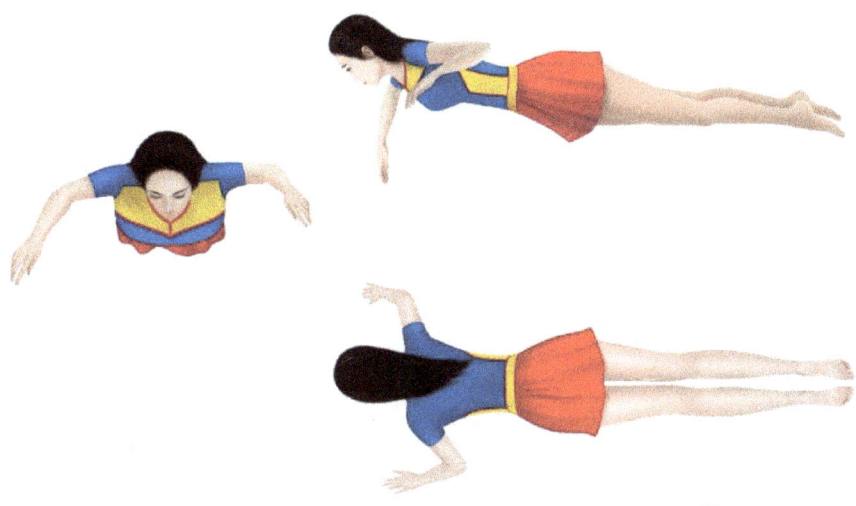

FIGURE 15

At this point, the right arm stroke has passed the 45° angle from the waterline. The strength of the stroke should diminish, following the angular acceleration chart in Appendix A, while the right arm stroke should be finishing to prepare for the next cycle. Your head has now completed its downward rotation, continuing to exhale. Meanwhile, the left arm is setting up for its stroke, with the upper arm positioned parallel to the waterline.

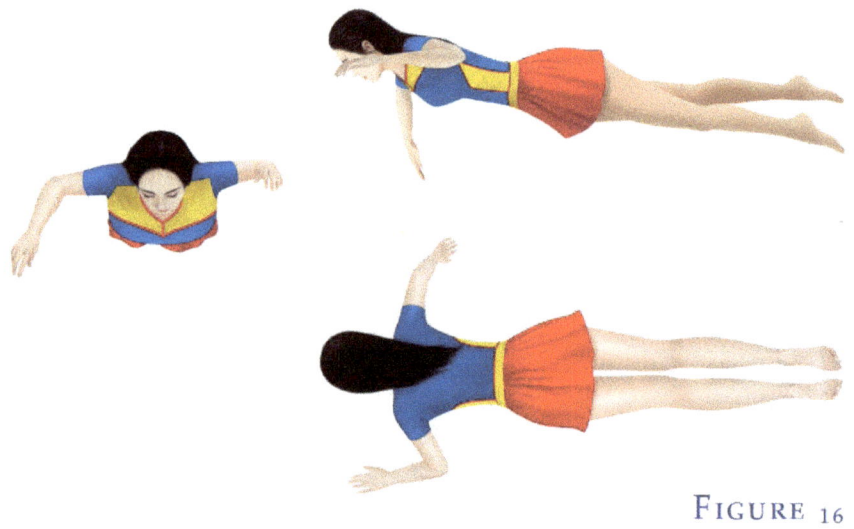

FIGURE 16

Once the right arm is slightly past the 90° angle and pointing downward, you should stop applying force to the stroke. It's time to begin lifting the right arm to prepare for the next stroke cycle. Notice that the left arm's forearm is parallel to and lightly grazing the water's surface. The arm shouldn't be fully underwater due to drag, nor should it be completely out of the water, as this would require extra energy to fight gravity. The optimal position for setting up the next stroke is one where the arm is just slightly touching the water's surface—not fully submerged nor entirely above it. This allows you to minimize drag while conserving energy by avoiding the need to lift the arm entirely out of the water.

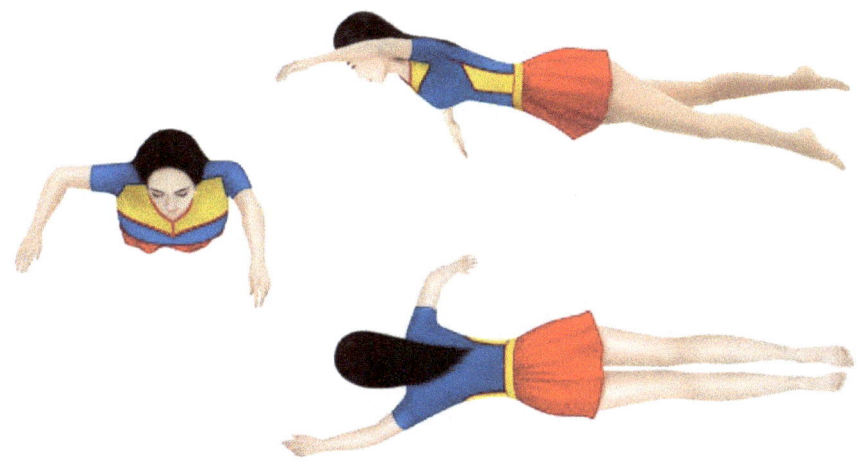

FIGURE 17

The right arm stroke should now be complete and ready to begin lifting for the next stroke cycle. Meanwhile, the left arm is positioned to start its stroke, stretched out in front with the hand just lightly grazing the water's surface—not fully above or submerged, to maximize efficiency. At this point, the head remains facing down in the water. The next step is to begin rotating the head upward to inhale and prepare for the next breath quickly.

Also, notice that we haven't focused on leg kicking. As mentioned earlier, kicking uses up to 75 percent more oxygen than an arm stroke, making it an inefficient constant motion. Instead, kicking should be purposeful, and used only when necessary to reposition or maintain balance. Of course, if a swimmer doesn't kick at all, their legs will likely sink, causing the body to tilt and potentially disrupt the swimming form.

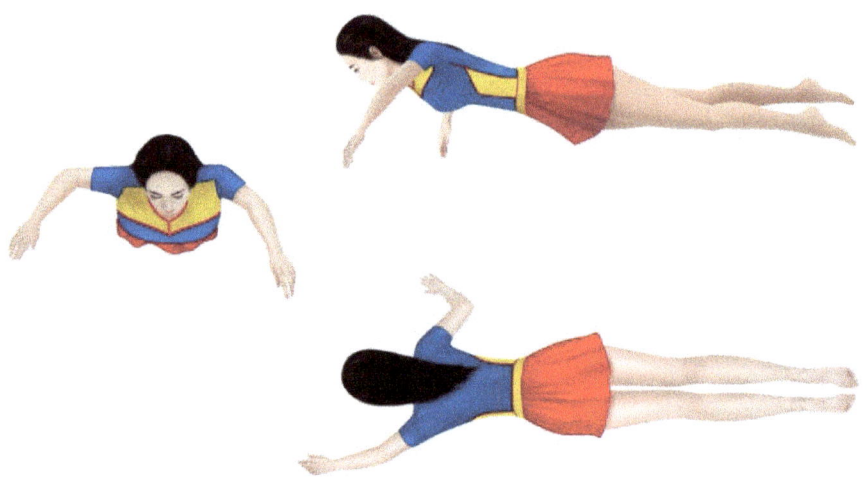

FIGURE 18

We've now completed one stroke with the right arm and one breathing cycle. Following the right arm stroke, the left arm will go through the same motion. At this point, the left arm is completing its stroke, similar to how the right arm did earlier. Meanwhile, the right arm, which just finished its stroke, is now slowly being lifted to set up for the next stroke.

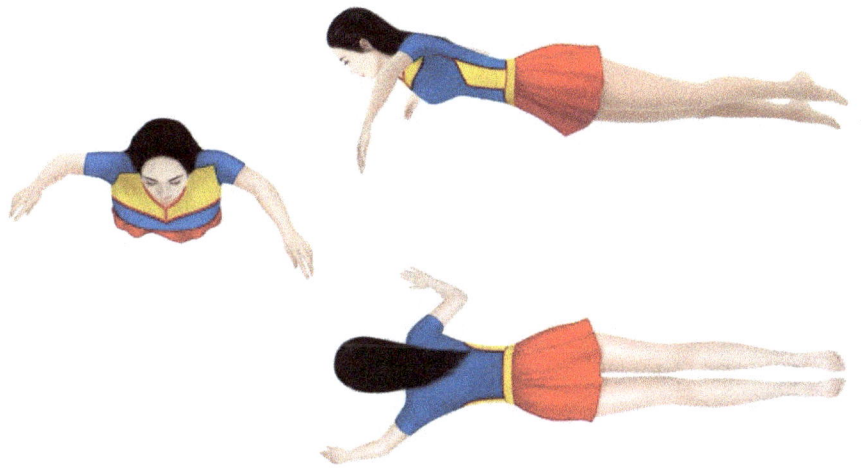

FIGURE 19

The left arm continues the stroke, and as it approaches 45°, the downward force should gradually decrease in line with the angular acceleration, preparing the arm to complete the stroke.

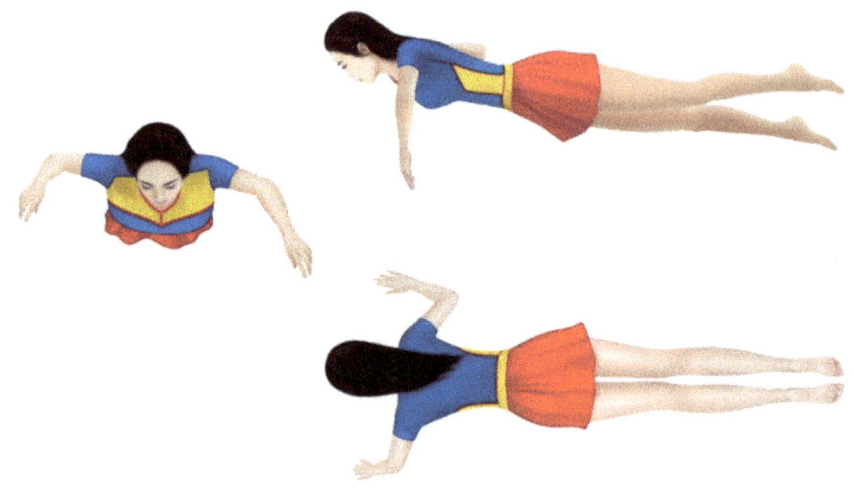

FIGURE 20

The left arm has now reached 90°, meaning all downward force for the stroke should cease. At this point, we've completed a full stroke cycle, with both the right and left arms stroking, along with one breathing cycle. Depending on your comfort level, you can choose to turn your head and breathe in every stroke cycle, as demonstrated here, or every two or three cycles. In rough ocean water, however, it may become necessary to breathe in every stroke cycle to maintain adequate oxygen.

Unlike other swimming techniques that prioritize speed, this technique focuses on comfort and leisure. With that in mind, the detailed movements outlined in this section serve as a foundational template. The key is to adapt and adjust these movements based on water conditions through improvisation. While fast-speed swimming techniques tend to be static and rigid, this technique is dynamic, making it especially well-suited for swimming in rough waters, where its full potential can be fully realized.

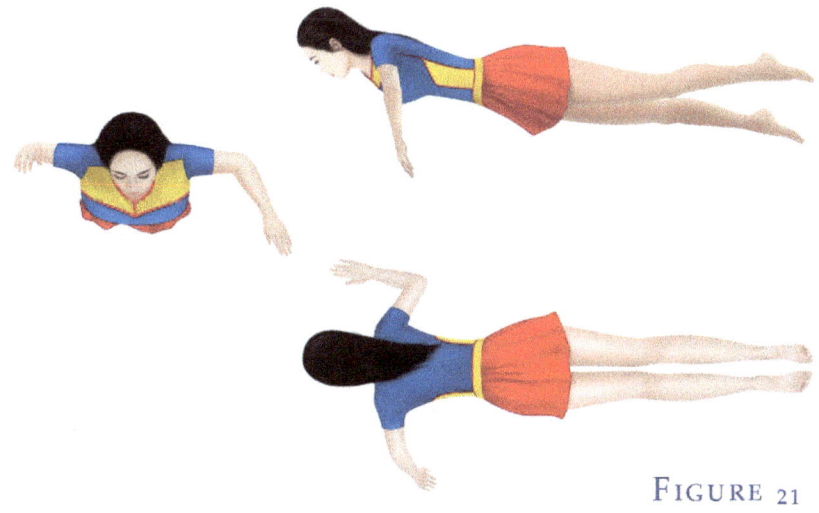

FIGURE 21

Pool Swimming

Start by entering the pool at one end and allow your body to adjust to the water temperature. Hold your breath and gently sink into the water, remaining submerged for about ten seconds. This brief acclimation period helps reduce the initial shock and prepares your body for better swimming performance.

First, assess your current swimming level and identify areas for improvement. Swim across the pool, then evaluate your performance. Were you able to make it across without stopping? If not, focus on refining your breathing and equilibrium techniques. If you completed the swim, can you swim back to finish a full lap? If not, breathing and equilibrium still need attention. The key takeaway is this: without proper breathing, no matter how good your strokes or kicks are, swimming becomes impossible. To truly master swimming, we must first master our breathing and pace.

If you can complete one full lap in the pool, it's time to shift focus to your swimming strokes. Keep in mind that kicking consumes an extra 75 percent of our oxygen[2], so we won't prioritize it here. Instead, focus on kicking for balance and positioning, while keeping your legs relatively straight to reduce drag. Revisiting the gravity-assisted swimming techniques and concepts from earlier will be beneficial as you move forward with this chapter.

Now, we can begin swimming across the pool using all the techniques described earlier. Start by standing at one end with your back against the wall. Remember in the previous chapter, the section on arm/elbow angles (Figures 5 and 6) showed a person sitting with their arm extended parallel to the floor in a relaxed position? Instead of sitting, you'll now be standing and doing the same thing. Extend your arm out naturally and relaxed, parallel to the water's surface, resting lightly on top of the water. This will be your starting position. From here, make a small hop off the pool floor, rising slightly to lie parallel to the water's surface, with your arm now resting on the water to begin swimming.

To begin swimming, use an elliptical pattern rotation with your arms. Your swimming strokes, breathing, and kicks should follow the techniques outlined in the detailed swimming movement section. All the necessary techniques have been thoroughly explained, providing you with enough knowledge to start swimming and learning on your own. With consistent practice, you'll gradually develop the ability to swim as fluidly and effortlessly as walking on land. Keep in mind this won't happen overnight—it requires years of dedication and refinement.

Fitness Test

To swim safely, it's essential to understand your current fitness level. Only by assessing your fitness can you confidently determine when it's safe to challenge yourself in rougher waters. There are several ways to assess swimming fitness, and we'll focus on two: the stair-stepping method and measuring how long you can swim continuously.

Stair-Stepping Test

The stair-stepping technique described refers to machine-aided stair-stepping, not using actual stairs. Like swimming, stair-stepping can provide a full-body workout, depending on how it's performed. Due to this similarity, it can serve as an effective fitness test for swimming. While stair-stepping can be challenging for beginners, don't be discouraged. Most beginners will initially be able to perform the stair-stepping method for ten to fifteen minutes, but with consistent practice, they can gradually build their endurance. The ultimate goal is to reach three hours.

Stair-Stepping Procedures

1. Make sure to bring plenty of water for the workout session.

2. Use an average-to-low speed setting on the step machine. The purpose is to do stair-stepping, not jogging.

3. Alternate the direction you face on the stair-stepper at different intervals. If your maximum session is eight minutes, alternate your stepping direction every two minutes, facing front, back, left, and right for two minutes each. If the session is forty minutes or more, alternate directions every ten minutes.

4. Use the center of strength to step. Combining the muscles of the entire body and stepping as one unit will reduce individual stress and result in prolonged workout sessions. This will also promote a full-body workout similar to swimming.

While using the arms for support during stair-stepping, the entire body's muscles should work together as one unit. The muscles must remain relaxed throughout the movement. Step as if there are eggshells beneath your feet—avoid stomping or making jarring, robotic movements. The motion should be fluid and continuous. Additionally, keep your knees slightly bent throughout all phases of the stair-stepping process. Ideally, stair-stepping should feel meditative, and by mastering this technique, we can gradually extend the session to reach our goal of three hours.

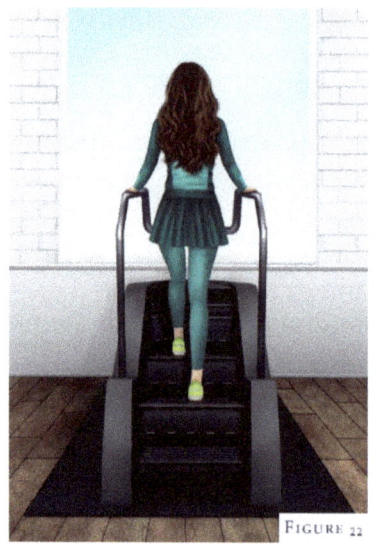

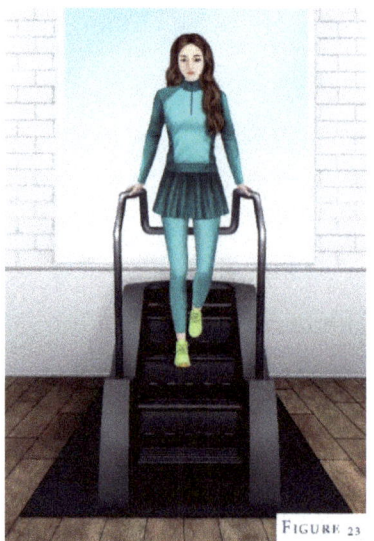

Step ten minutes facing forward.

Step ten minutes facing backward.

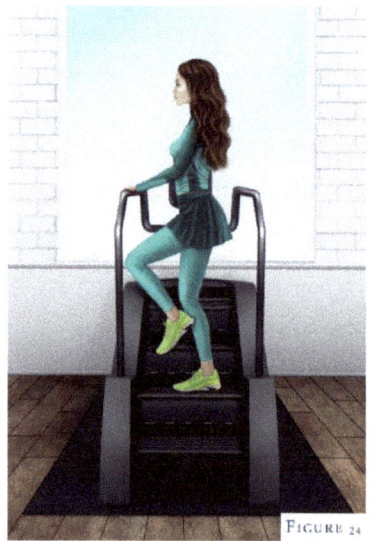

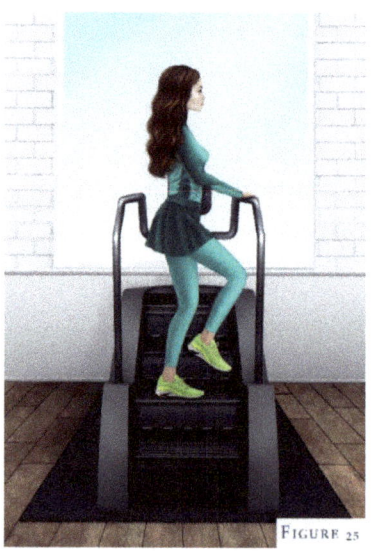

Step ten minutes facing left.

Step ten minutes facing right.
Repeat by facing forward again.

Swimming Test

The second fitness test measures swimming endurance. You should aim to swim continuously for at least three hours in the pool without feeling out of breath. Once you can swim for three hours without fatigue, you'll have the endurance needed for more challenging environments. After passing both the stair-stepping and swimming tests, you'll be prepared to handle rougher waters outside of a pool.

Ocean Swimming

Swimming in the ocean presents risks, such as encounters with marine life and challenging conditions like rip currents. Before proceeding with this chapter, ensure that you have mastered all the previous topics in this book and have passed the fitness test. Always follow safety guidelines and heed any advice from local beach authorities. Only swim within the view of a lifeguard.

Contrary to popular belief, the farther out from the shore you swim, the easier it can be due to the absence of waves crashing against the beach. The area where the waves crash is the toughest to swim in, as it's the roughest. However, this also presents the greatest challenge and fun for advanced swimmers. If you're a beginner, start by swimming only at beaches with lifeguards on duty and under green flag conditions, indicating calm water. For safety reasons, never swim farther than knee-deep from the shore or in rough water conditions.

The first step at the beach is to assess the direction of the ocean's current, as this is crucial if you need to swim to safety. To do this, find a dry twig or leaf and throw it into the water. The direction the object moves indicates the flow of the current. Please be aware that the current can change depending on the tides. Identify prominent landmarks along the shore to use as reference points while swimming. Always check that the water is calm, with no rough waves, strong winds, or powerful currents. Ensure your goggles are clean and fog-free for a clear view. Begin by wading out, staying aware of the current, and once the water reaches knee-depth, start swimming.

Air management is critical while swimming, especially in the ocean. Breathing is considerably more challenging when navigating rough waves than when swimming in a pool. In the pool, you can establish a rhythm—breathing, for example, every third stroke—to maintain a smooth and efficient stroke pattern. But in the ocean, you have to take advantage of any opening to breathe, depending on the conditions of the water. When waves are crashing frequently, it's even more crucial to carefully time your breathing. Remember the equilibrium technique: you're not racing anyone, so if you're struggling to breathe, it's important to slow down. Your swimming session will end when you run out of air. To avoid this, maintain a steady swimming pace and employ the equilibrium technique to sustain your efforts.

Swimming in crashing waves is an entirely different experience compared to swimming in a pool. Unlike in calm water, we don't completely ignore the waves but learn to adjust to them. When a wave hits, we can keep swimming through it, allowing the water to rise and fall around us as we maintain our stroke. However, it's important to anticipate the wave before it arrives. Assess whether you'll have time for another breath and how powerful the wave will be. If it's a small wave, you can continue swimming as usual. But if the wave is stronger, turn to face it at a 90° angle, lowering your head. As the wave approaches, stop swimming and relax, allowing it to pass over you. Once it's gone, resume swimming parallel to the shore again.

Breathing can be challenging when waves crash against you. A useful solution is to adjust your head position when you turn to breathe. Instead of turning your head completely sideways or facing forward, angle your face slightly toward your shoulder. This way, your nose and mouth are less likely to be hit by the incoming waves, making it easier to take a breath.

At times, it's necessary to reduce your stroke or even stop stroking entirely if a wave hits you. Occasionally, the wave may be so large that raising your arm above it becomes impossible. Swimming in the ocean is about seizing opportunities. You stroke when you can, and you breathe when the moment allows. The key is to avoid getting winded and to maintain a steady pace throughout.

All the techniques discussed earlier—gravity-assisted swimming, equilibrium, swimming like a fish riddle, proper strokes, and breathing—must be mastered before attempting ocean swimming. While beach swimming is a fun and rewarding experience, it can also be dangerous. It requires years of practice and refinement before you should even consider venturing into the ocean. Stay safe, enjoy the journey, and have fun while practicing your skills.

CHAPTER V

Swimming Riddle Answer

If you want to swim like a fish,

think like a fish.

If you want to think like a fish,

think like a human.

If you can swim without a care

As if the water is not there

Riding the waves but half asleep

Like any fish in ocean's deep

The answer to this riddle holds the key to swimming like a fish. Once we adopt the mindset of a fish while swimming, we can glide through the water as effortlessly as walking on land. To solve this riddle, we must carefully analyze the clues in each sentence and then work backward to uncover the solution.

If you want to swim like a fish,
think like a fish.

To swim like a fish, we must first think like one. However, as humans, it's impossible for us to truly think like a fish. While we understand that thinking like a fish would enable us to swim like one, it's both mentally and physically beyond our reach. This is where the second part of the riddle comes in, offering us further clues to help us achieve this goal.

If you want to think like a fish,
think like a human.

We can accept the second part of the riddle because, as humans, we can think like ourselves. While we may never fully understand a fish's thought processes, we can use deductive reasoning to work backward and solve the first part of the riddle. How do humans approach swimming in ways that differ from fish? To answer this question, we must first ask ourselves another:

What similarities do fish and humans share in swimming—physically, mentally, and environmentally?

If we trust in science and evolutionary processes, we'd need to look millions of years back to compare human and fish anatomy, so physical similarities can be ruled out. Since we're humans and can't think like a fish mentally, we can only use deductive reasoning. That leaves us with the environmental aspect as a basis for comparison. Fish live in water, while humans are surrounded by air on land. With this, we can proceed with our reasoning to solve the riddle.

Atmospheric pressure at sea level on Earth is about 14.7 pounds per square inch[4]. For most of our lives, we're unaware of the air around us, despite it pressing on us from all directions. Air is so natural to us that we don't see it and tend to ignore it in our daily activities. This is how humans relate to air: we don't consciously think about it. Similarly, by understanding this, we can infer that a fish perceives the water in the same way. Just as we don't notice the air around us, a fish doesn't notice the water it swims through. A fish swims effortlessly because water is second nature to it. In the same way, humans carry out their daily routines while subconsciously ignoring the air around them, much like how fish ignore the water.

So, how do we swim like a fish? We swim like a fish by learning to ignore the water, too! Just as we walk through the air without consciously noticing it, we should swim by feel, not by sight. When we walk from point A to point B, we don't focus on the air around us, even though it's pressing on us from all sides. If there's a strong wind blowing against us, we adjust by leaning into it, but we continue walking forward. Similarly, when swimming, we go through the motions of the stroke and adjust to the water's conditions. The key is to move fluidly, without overthinking or fighting the water.

Using this analogy, we can also ignore the water while swimming. Just as we don't consciously focus on the air around us while walking, we can ignore the water itself as we go through the motion of swimming. However, just like feeling the wind when it blows against us, we must adjust to the water conditions. The goal is to move fluidly through the water, responding to its changes without letting it disrupt our rhythm. Below are several scenarios that will help clarify this concept further.

The goal is to swim in a way that we're so attuned to the water that we don't consciously think about it as if we're sleeping. Just like we don't think about the air around us while walking, we want to swim with the same level of ease, fluidity, and naturalness. Even though the water is still there, it becomes secondary to the motion of swimming itself. When we reach that point, we're effectively moving through the water without being obstructed or slowed down by it. The water becomes just another medium we move through, much like walking through air. That's when we truly swim like a fish—effortlessly and in harmony with the water.

It's ironic, but the less we focus on the water, the easier swimming becomes. To help clarify this concept, let's consider a few examples of what it means to "ignore" the water. Take a TV, for instance. When it's turned off and we're sitting on the sofa, all we see is a regular, unremarkable TV. But once the TV starts playing our favorite movie, we stop seeing the TV itself and become completely absorbed in the film. The TV ceases to exist in our minds at that moment because we're not focused on the object itself; we're immersed in what it's showing us. Similarly, when we swim, the key is to stop fixating on the water and instead immerse ourselves in the experience of swimming.

Another analogy can be drawn from hidden 3D images. To see the 3D image, we must first ignore the distracting, random patterns that make up the background. Once we train our focus and recognize the 3D figure, the chaotic patterns disappear from our perception, and all we can see is the hidden image. Similarly, in swimming, once we stop focusing on the water itself we can move through it effortlessly. Below is an example of a hidden 3D image—notice the lady swimming toward the left.

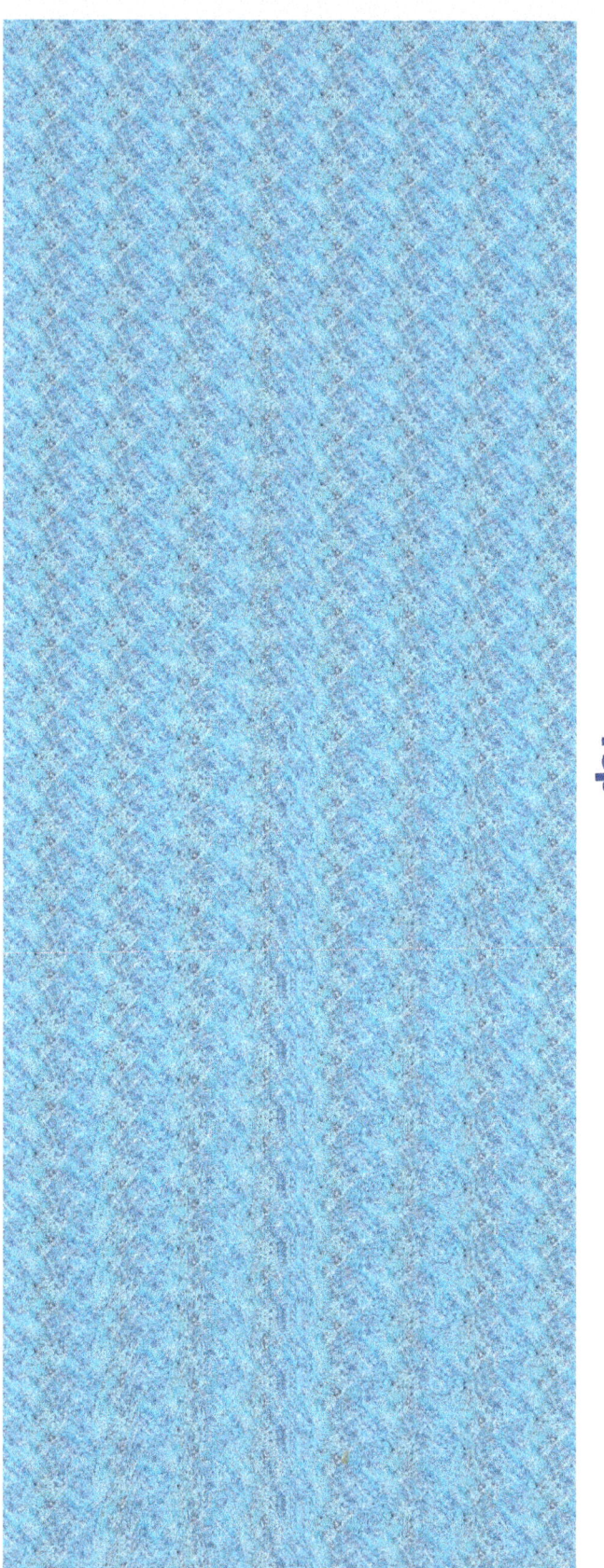

Top

If we jump into the water and view it simply as water, we won't swim as effectively as we might expect. Instead, we need to move beyond simply seeing the water and focus on feeling it. Yes, the water will create pressure against us and move around us, but if we can ignore these sensations and instead tune into the natural ebb and flow, we can react to it instinctively. By swimming with the water, rather than against it, we'll become more in sync with the environment, making our strokes smoother and more efficient.

Water is never static; it's constantly shifting and changing. As such, our swim strokes must also adapt in response to these fluctuations. Our technique should be flexible, adjusting in real-time to the water conditions by anticipating and adapting to them. Rather than fighting against the water, we should flow with it, working with its rhythm and energy to maximize efficiency.

Consider a fishing bobber—does it have any awareness of the water, or is the water aware of the bobber? If both the bobber and the water were to ignore each other, how could the bobber float so effortlessly? The answer lies in the bobber's intrinsic properties. It floats naturally because it doesn't focus on the water; instead, it works with the water's natural buoyancy, maintaining its position effortlessly without any conscious effort. Similarly, by working with the water's natural flow, we too can swim with ease.

Since the overall density of humans is less than that of water, we should be able to achieve the same effortless motion as a fishing bobber by ignoring the water itself. The water isn't aware of us, and we shouldn't focus on it either—except for the natural sensations of pressure, ebb, and flow. By harnessing the water's inherent properties, we can react dynamically and adjust our swimming techniques to adapt to the constantly changing conditions. This way, one swims in harmony with the water's natural movements.

Imagine a fish swimming in a pond. If we make a sound while walking nearby, the fish will scatter and hide. To the fish, the water is like a spider's web—it can every vibration, no matter how faint. We should not treat water as an obstacle to overcome; instead, we should think of it as an extension of our senses extending outward like the web of a spider. Much like the fish, we should aim to feel every single molecule of water around us. When we feel the water rushing toward us, we can then adjust and swim with it, not against it.

Swimming techniques are typically static, but the water is always in motion, especially in rough conditions. Instead of using the same swim stroke to fight the water, adopt a dynamic stroke that adjusts to the ever-changing water conditions. Feel the ebb and flow of the water, and modify your strokes accordingly. Swim as if walking on land—smoothly and naturally. Reduce your awareness of the water and minimize the shock factor, which occurs when you're exposed to an environment that feels vastly different from your current surroundings. By adapting in this way, you'll swim more fluidly and efficiently.

For the final analogy, let's explore the shock factor —the sudden sensation we experience when jumping into a body of water from dry land. To swim effortlessly, or as some refer to it, to "immerse" ourselves in the water, we must reduce this shock factor to zero. To better illustrate this, we can use an analogy from outer space. Imagine the transition from the comfort of gravity on land to the sensation of weightlessness in space. Just as astronauts adapt to the absence of gravity, we need to adjust to the water environment by embracing it fully and minimizing the initial shock.

Imagine a blob floating in outer space, completely weightless. One day, it stumbles upon a teleportation device and beams down to Earth. The moment it arrives, what's the first thing it says? The truth is, it can't say anything at all, because it's instantly squashed by the overwhelming force of gravity and air pressure. In this scenario, the shock factor is 100 percent and cannot be mitigated, as it is completely unprepared for the drastic change in the Earth's environment.

Fortunately, jumping into a body of water from dry land isn't quite like a blob being beamed to Earth from outer space. While the shock factor isn't as extreme as it would be for the blob, it's still significant. This is why some people panic, thrash around, and struggle to swim—even when their lives depend on it— after jumping into the water. The sudden immersion can be overwhelming, triggering a fight-or-flight response, and they may forget the techniques needed to stay calm and swim efficiently.

Our goal is to reduce the shock factor to zero percent. Instead of treating water as an obstacle or a force to overcome, we should view it as a tool or medium that we swim through. The shock factor leads us to a swimming paradox: People can swim because there's water; yet, people can't swim because they think they're swimming in water. The paradox lies in that simple shift of perspective—once we stop focusing on the water as something separate and start integrating it as a part of our natural swimming movement, we can swim more effortlessly.

To swim as effortlessly as if we're sleeping or as a fish, we need to blur the fine line where the air and water meet until we can't tell the difference anymore. Once we treat the water we swim in as if we're walking on land, we gain complete control over it. Our breathing becomes just as controlled as it is on land, meaning we won't feel tired or winded while swimming. Ultimately, this will allow us to swim as naturally as a fish in its environment—effortless, fluid, and in perfect harmony with the water.

Anticipated Questions

Where did the swimming technique and swimming riddle come from?

The swimming riddle and techniques described in this book are unique to my approach. If they happen to resemble anything found elsewhere, it is purely coincidental. I have not learned this from any other sources, but have instead developed it through years of self-teaching, trial and error, and reflection on my personal experiences with swimming.

How long does it take to master this swimming technique?

Everyone's experience is different. Some will learn to swim faster than others. I spent over ten years swimming in both the pool and the ocean before mastering this technique.

What are the benefits of mastering this technique?

By mastering the techniques of equilibrium, gravity-assisted swimming, and adapting to the water's flow, we're not just improving our ability to swim longer or more effortlessly but also ensuring that we can handle challenging situations like rip currents. By staying calm and leveraging our technique, we can respond to natural forces instead of fighting against them, ultimately making us safer to swim in rough waters.

What are the drawbacks of mastering this technique?

It is highly recommended that swimmers avoid seeking out rough or dangerous water conditions. If you do swim in such conditions, people might mistakenly call 911 to try to save you, assuming that if the water is that rough, someone can't swim in it. I've personally had 911 called on me twice, involving lifeguards and ambulances, even though I was swimming normally at the beach. I've also been approached by the Coast Guard to check if I needed help while swimming. Those 911 calls left me shaken, and now I'm hesitant to swim in rough water, as it often results in lifeguards taking unnecessary risks to "save" me when I don't need saving.

Conclusion

A lot of valuable insights were covered in this book, and it's understandable if you feel overwhelmed or like you've missed something. Don't expect to swim effortlessly right after reading this book—mastery takes time. For me, it took six years to swim comfortably in the pool and ten years to feel at ease in the ocean. I've experienced many trials and errors along the way, and I hope this book helps you avoid some of the same struggles I faced. Patience, practice, and dedication will be your best tools in the journey ahead.

Swimming is as much a mental challenge as a physical one. If we see ourselves as merely moving through water, we impose limits on ourselves—losing half the battle before we even begin. Just as we move through air effortlessly without a second thought, a fish glides through water with the same ease. By shifting our mindset and breaking free from the notion that water is an obstacle, we can transcend its constraints. When the boundary between air and water dissolves in our minds, we gain full control over our movements, adapting effortlessly to any conditions—even the roughest waters. Swim as if the water isn't there, and you'll move through it with ease.

Mastering proper breathing is far more crucial than perfecting strokes or kicks. If there's only one swimming skill to focus on, it should be breathing—because without air, swimming becomes impossible. Pace yourself and apply the equilibrium technique. Leverage gravity to work with you, not against you. Stay relaxed and engage your muscles as a unified system rather than in isolated movements. Develop an understanding of angular acceleration to execute fluid, efficient swim strokes. With these principles, swimming becomes effortless and sustainable.

Water patterns are infinite, making it impossible to conquer them with rigid, finite techniques. This is especially true when swimming in the ocean's surf, where waves crash unpredictably. Many skilled swimmers struggle in these conditions because they rely on a streamlined technique designed for speed in calm water. To navigate rough water effectively, especially at the beach, you must adapt your swimming style to the ever-changing environment. Anticipate the water's movement and adjust before the next wave hits. Continuously feel and respond to the shifting conditions. True mastery comes not from fighting the water but from working with it.

Most importantly, always prioritize safety. Swim only in areas monitored by lifeguards and within water conditions that match your comfort and skill level. No technique or experience can replace caution and good judgment. The ocean is unpredictable, and even the strongest swimmers must respect its power. Stay aware, trust your instincts, and never take unnecessary risks.

APPENDIX A
Effect of Gravity
While Swimming

The Gravity-Assisted Swimming (GAS) method takes advantage of natural forces to optimize swimming efficiency. Since our arms swing at the shoulder like a hinged rod, we can analyze them as rotating on a frictionless pivot to determine the most effective way to harness gravity while swimming. Even though the human arm is not a perfectly uniform rod, this model helps us understand how to execute a swimming stroke that maximizes the benefits of gravity and angular acceleration. By aligning our movements with these principles, we can reduce energy expenditure, improve stroke efficiency, and swim with greater ease.

If the rod is released from rest at an angle beneath the horizon, what is the angular acceleration of the rod immediately after it is released?

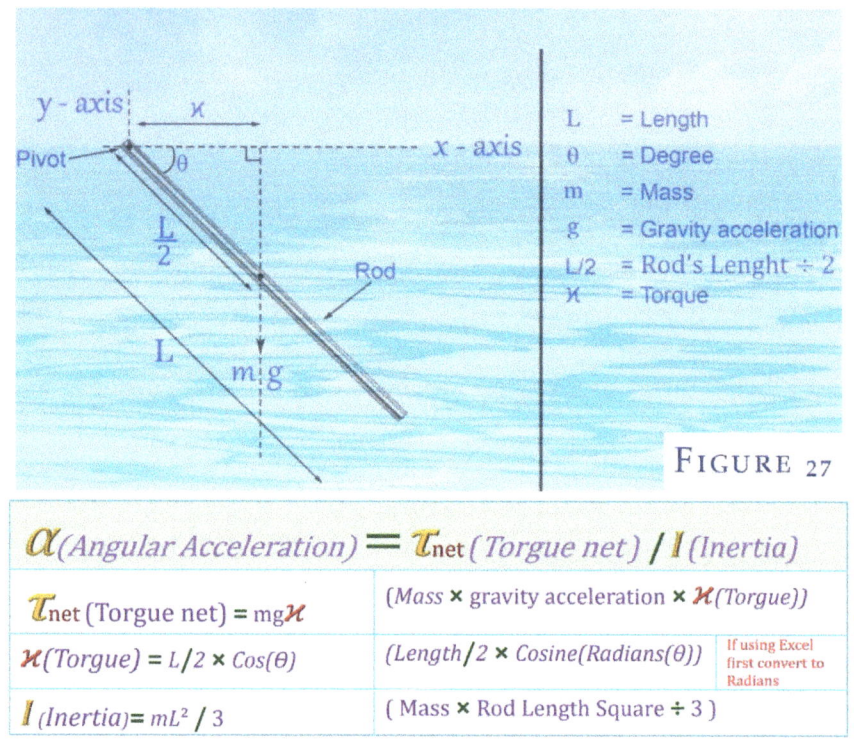

FIGURE 27

α (Angular Acceleration) $= \tau_{net}$ (Torgue net) $/ I$ (Inertia)		
τ_{net} (Torgue net) $= mg\varkappa$	(Mass × gravity acceleration × $\varkappa$(Torque))	
$\varkappa$(Torque) $= L/2 × Cos(\theta)$	(Length/2 × Cosine(Radians(θ))	If using Excel first convert to Radians
I (Inertia)$= mL^2 / 3$	(Mass × Rod Length Square ÷ 3)	

FIGURE 28

We have the length **L**, mass **m**, gravity acceleration **g**, and degree of the angle θ similar to our arm angle below the water line when we stroke. Using these values and the angular acceleration equation, we can calculate the best approach to swimming by stroking. First, we use length **L** divided by 2 multiplied by the cosine of the radian(θ) to get torque $\varkappa$. Using mass **m** multiplied by gravity acceleration g multiplied by torque ϰ, we get torque net τnet. Using

mass m multiplied by length **L** squared and then divided by 3, we get

inertia *I*. Using torque net τnet divided by inertia *I*, we get angular

acceleration α. Using these formulas, we plot the values in the table for

360° as shown.

g	m	L	L/2	θ	ϰ	τ_{net}	I	α
Gravity	Mass	Rod's Length	Rod's Length / 2	Degree	Torque	Torque Net	Inertia	Angular Acceleration
meter/s²	kg	meter	meter	θ	L/2(Cos(θ))	mgϰ	mL²/3	τnet/I
9.81	5	1	0.5	0	0.5000	24.5250	1.6667	14.72
9.81	5	1	0.5	10	0.4924	24.1524	1.6667	14.49
9.81	5	1	0.5	20	0.4698	23.0460	1.6667	13.83
9.81	5	1	0.5	30	0.4330	21.2393	1.6667	12.74
9.81	5	1	0.5	40	0.3830	18.7872	1.6667	11.27
9.81	5	1	0.5	50	0.3214	15.7644	1.6667	9.46
9.81	5	1	0.5	60	0.2500	12.2625	1.6667	7.36
9.81	5	1	0.5	70	0.1710	8.3880	1.6667	5.03
9.81	5	1	0.5	80	0.0868	4.2587	1.6667	2.56
9.81	5	1	0.5	90	0.0000	0.0000	1.6667	0.00
9.81	5	1	0.5	100	-0.0868	-4.2587	1.6667	-2.56
9.81	5	1	0.5	110	-0.1710	-8.3880	1.6667	-5.03
9.81	5	1	0.5	120	-0.2500	-12.2625	1.6667	-7.36
9.81	5	1	0.5	130	-0.3214	-15.7644	1.6667	-9.46
9.81	5	1	0.5	140	-0.3830	-18.7872	1.6667	-11.27
9.81	5	1	0.5	150	-0.4330	-21.2393	1.6667	-12.74
9.81	5	1	0.5	160	-0.4698	-23.0460	1.6667	-13.83
9.81	5	1	0.5	170	-0.4924	-24.1524	1.6667	-14.49
9.81	5	1	0.5	180	-0.5000	-24.5250	1.6667	-14.72
9.81	5	1	0.5	190	-0.4924	-24.1524	1.6667	-14.49
9.81	5	1	0.5	200	-0.4698	-23.0460	1.6667	-13.83
9.81	5	1	0.5	210	-0.4330	-21.2393	1.6667	-12.74
9.81	5	1	0.5	220	-0.3830	-18.7872	1.6667	-11.27
9.81	5	1	0.5	230	-0.3214	-15.7644	1.6667	-9.46
9.81	5	1	0.5	240	-0.2500	-12.2625	1.6667	-7.36
9.81	5	1	0.5	250	-0.1710	-8.3880	1.6667	-5.03
9.81	5	1	0.5	260	-0.0868	-4.2587	1.6667	-2.56
9.81	5	1	0.5	270	0.0000	0.0000	1.6667	0.00
9.81	5	1	0.5	280	0.0868	4.2587	1.6667	2.56
9.81	5	1	0.5	290	0.1710	8.3880	1.6667	5.03
9.81	5	1	0.5	300	0.2500	12.2625	1.6667	7.36
9.81	5	1	0.5	310	0.3214	15.7644	1.6667	9.46
9.81	5	1	0.5	320	0.3830	18.7872	1.6667	11.27
9.81	5	1	0.5	330	0.4330	21.2393	1.6667	12.74
9.81	5	1	0.5	340	0.4698	23.0460	1.6667	13.83
9.81	5	1	0.5	350	0.4924	24.1524	1.6667	14.49
9.81	5	1	0.5	360	0.5000	24.5250	1.6667	14.72

FIGURE 29

Using the calculated values above for angular acceleration,we plot them in a series of charts labeled as Return on Effort Per Swim Stroke.

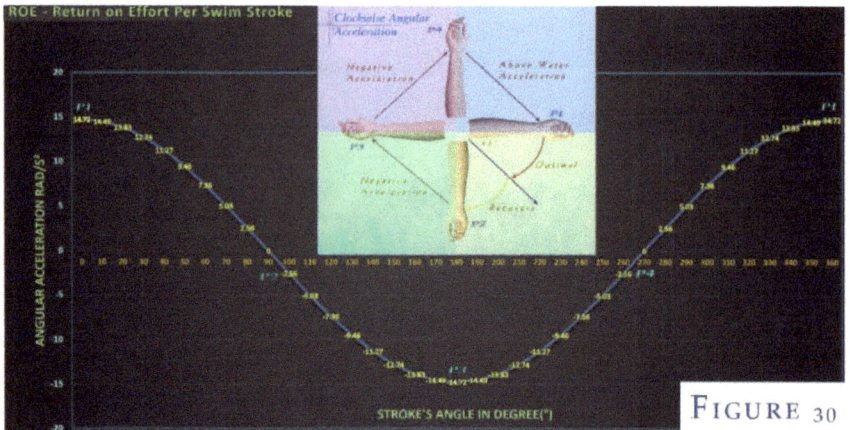

FIGURE 30

The X-axis represents the stroke angle relative to the front waterline, measured in degrees and rotating clockwise. These values are displayed horizontally in orange at the middle of the chart. The Y-axis represents the calculated angular acceleration, derived from the table above, and is shown vertically in blue on the left side of the chart. For easier analysis, the corresponding angular acceleration values are also displayed in yellow along the curve. Additionally, an image is plotted in the top-middle section of the chart, illustrating the full 360° motion divided into four quadrants. This visual representation helps in understanding how stroke angles and angular acceleration interact to optimize swimming efficiency.

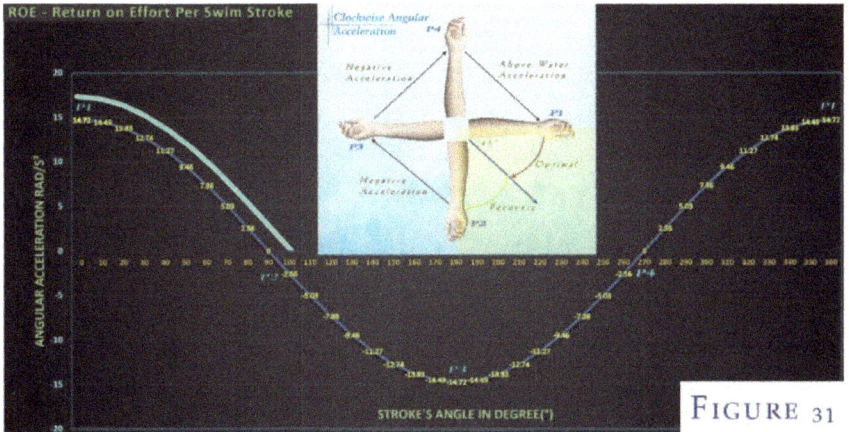

FIGURE 31

The first quadrant, from P1 to P2, is shaded yellow and represents the initial phase of a normal swimming stroke. It begins at 0°, when the arm is extended forward, parallel to the waterline, and making contact with the water. The stroke then moves downward to 90°, where the arm points straight down toward the bottom. During this phase, the angular acceleration starts at its highest value of 14.72 rad/s² when the arm is fully extended and resting on the waterline. As the stroke progresses and the arm moves downward, the angular acceleration gradually decreases, reaching its lowest point when the arm is perpendicular to the waterline at 90°. This phase is crucial for generating propulsion while maintaining efficiency in stroke mechanics.

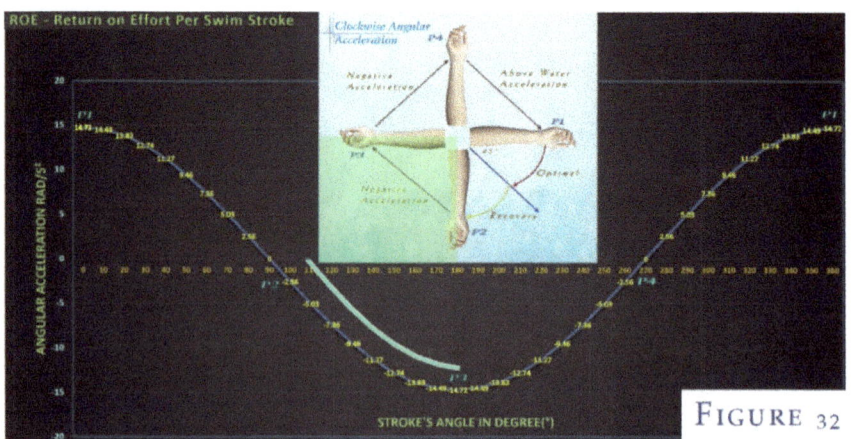

FIGURE 32

The second quadrant, from P2 to P3 and shaded green, begins when the arm is pointing straight down at 90° and continues stroking backward past the waist toward the legs. Since this movement is directed upward, it works against gravity, resulting in negative angular acceleration.

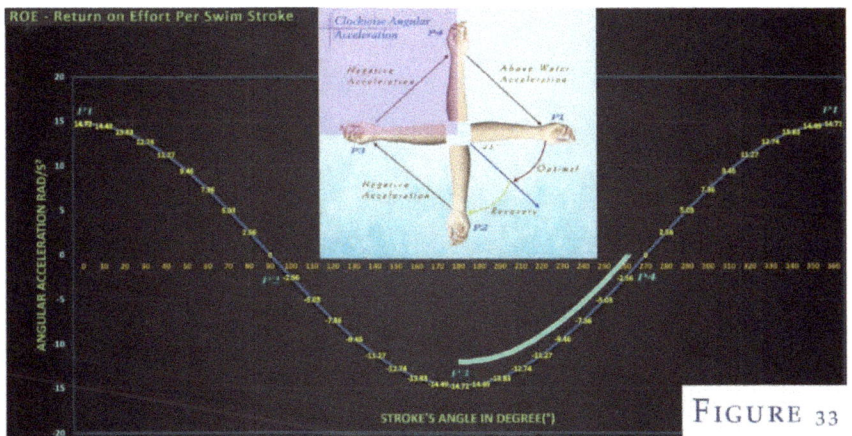

FIGURE 33

The third quadrant, from P3 to P4 and shaded purple, begins when the arm is extended straight behind the waist at 180°, moving upward toward the sky. This motion is physically impossible for most people and works against gravity, resulting in negative angular acceleration.

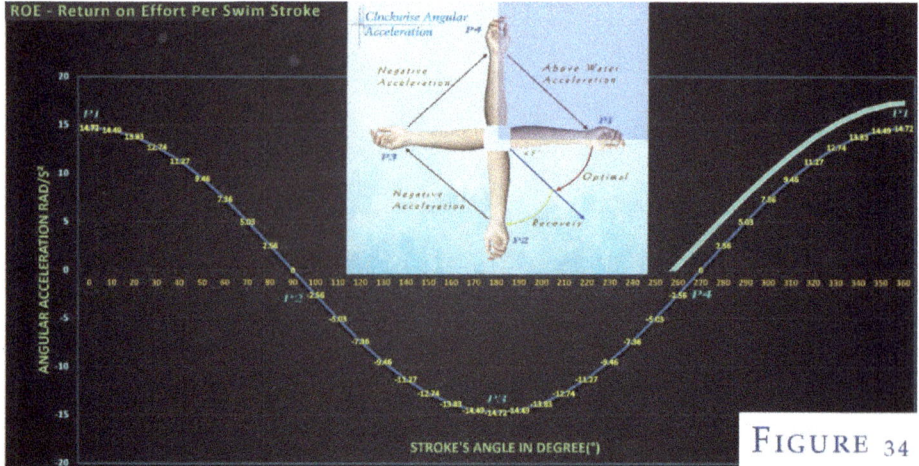

FIGURE 34

The fourth quadrant from P4 to P1 is shaded as blue and starts by pointing straight up at the sky at 270°, stroking down to the water's surface.

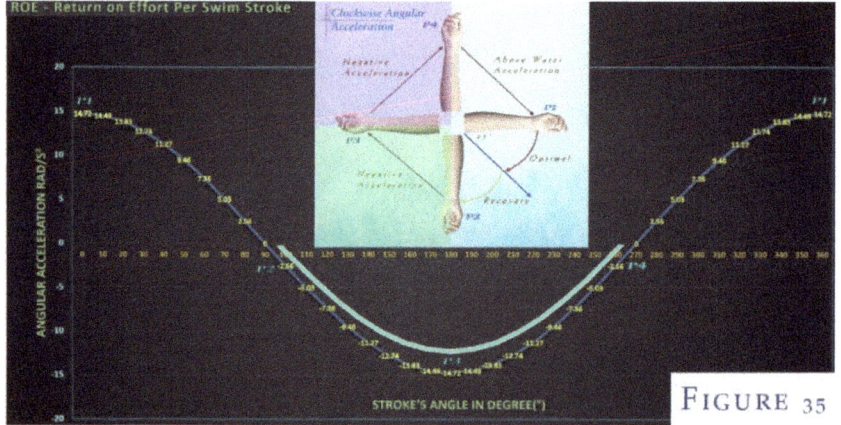

FIGURE 35

Since the quadrants from P2 to P3 (green) and P3 to P4 (purple) are both negative angular accelerations, they're removed from consideration for optimal swim stroke.

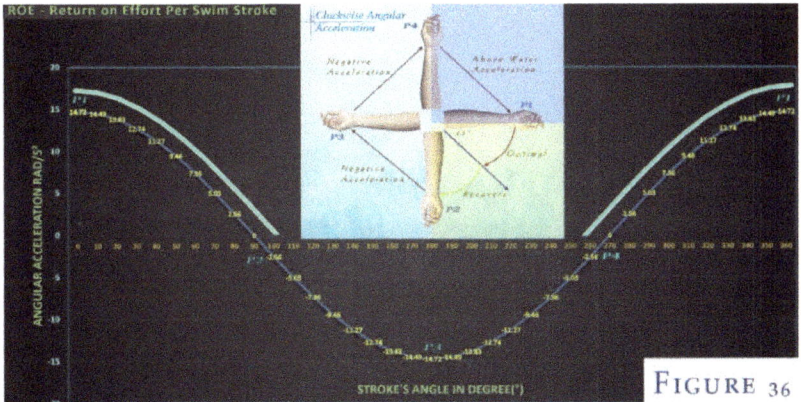

FIGURE 36

This leaves us with the quadrants from P1 to P2 (yellow) and P4 to P1 (blue), both exhibiting positive angular acceleration, which are key considerations for an optimal swimming stroke.

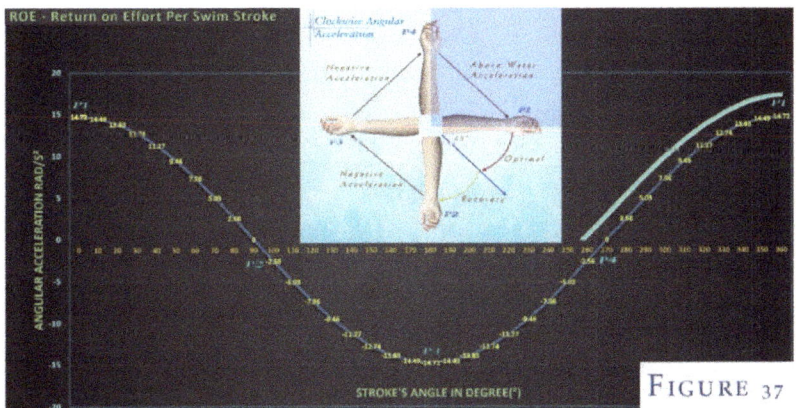

FIGURE 37

Since the quadrant from P4 to P1 (blue), starting at 270° and pointing straight up, involves stroking through empty air before slapping the water at P1, there is no propulsion generated from the arm's contact with the water. Additionally, raising the arm to the P4 position requires fighting gravity, further reducing swimming efficiency.

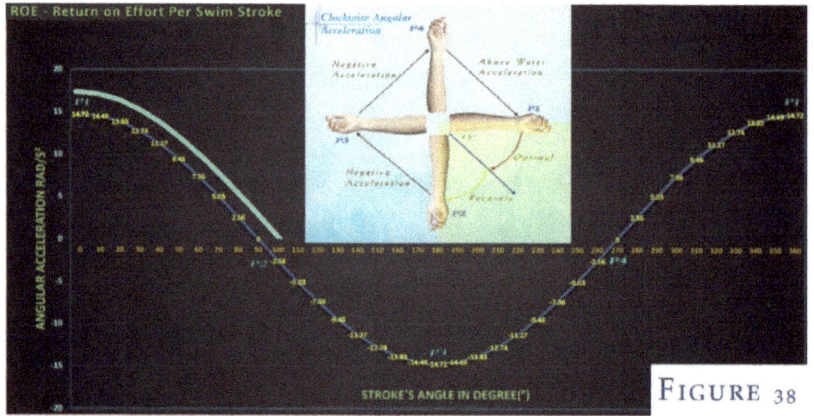

FIGURE 38

This leaves only one optimal quadrant, from P1 to P2 (yellow), starting at 0°, where the arm points forward. The angular acceleration is highest when the arm is parallel to the waterline at 0°. As the stroke progresses toward P2 (90° downward), the angular acceleration decreases, with diminishing returns as we approach P2, where the arm points straight down.

To perform the most optimal stroke and maximize the use of gravity, we need to finish the stroke at around a 45° angle below the waterline. At this point, bring the arm up for the next stroke. The goal of the swimming technique in this book is not to swim fast, but to swim as if you're sleeping—efficiently and relaxed. The optimal use of gravity provides the most efficient and restful swim stroke. Techniques designed to maximize speed, using extreme or rapid strokes, are not the focus here. While some swimming techniques may involve stroking past 45° for speed, that's not the aim of this approach.

References

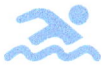

1. **Centers for Disease Control and Prevention (CDC)**

http://www.cdc.gov

2. **Oxygen Use of Freestyle Kicks – Adrian 1966.**

https://blog.arenaswim.com/us/training-technique-us/science-swimming-mysteries-freestyle-leg-kick/

3. **Arm Weight**

https://exrx.net/Kinesiology/Segments

4. **Atmospheric Pressure**

https://www.britannica.com/science/atmospheric-pressure

5. **Contribution Of Arm Stroke And Leg Kick To Freestyle Swimming**

https://bms.sport-iat.de/Record/4032609

Morris, K. S., Skinner, T. L., Jenkins, D. G., Osborne, M., Shephard, M. E.

About the Author

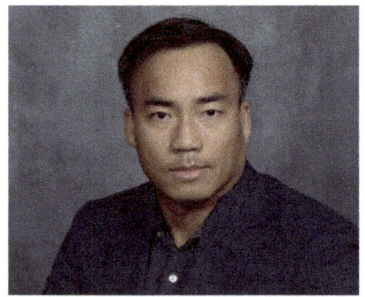

Alex Natare was born in Vung Tau, Vietnam. He immigrated to the USA and has lived in Virginia, New York, and Texas, and now resides in Florida.